Current Nursing Practice titles

Already published

Accident and Emergency Nursing
Ear, Nose and Throat Nursing
Neuromedical and Neurosurgical Nursing
Plastic Surgical and Burns Nursing
Applied Nutrition and Dietetics
Stoma Care Nursing

In preparation

Gastroenterological Nursing

Ophthalmic Nursing

Mary Kirton RGN, OND

Sister
Casualty and Out-patients Department
Glasgow Eye Infirmary, Glasgow

Marion Richardson BD, SRN, RCNT, DN (Lond.)

Formerly Clinical Teacher
Accident and Emergency Department
St Thomas' Hospital, London

Third Edition

Baillière Tindall
London Philadelphia Toronto Sydney Tokyo

Baillière Tindall 24–28 Oval Road
W.B. Saunders London NW1 7DX

West Washington Square
Philadelphia, PA 19105, USA

1 Goldthorne Avenue
Toronto, Ontario M8Z 5T9, Canada

ABP Australia Ltd
44–50 Waterloo Road
North Ryde, NSW 2113, Australia

Harcourt Brace Jovanovich Japan Inc
Ichibancho Central Building, 22–1 Ichibancho
Chiyoda-ku, Tokyo 102, Japan

First published 1975
Second edition 1981
Third edition 1987

Typeset by Photographics, Honiton, Devon
Printed in Great Britain at the Alden Press, Oxford

British Library Cataloguing in Publication Data

Kirton Mary
    Ophthalmic nursing — 3rd ed. —
    (Current nursing practice).
    1. Ophthalmic nursing 2. Eye — Diseases and defects
    I. Title II. Richardson, Marion
    III. Darling, Vera IV. Series
    617.7′0024613   RE88

ISBN 0–7020–1254–8

Contents

Preface

'The light of the body is the eye.' Matthew 6:22.

Nursing patients with ophthalmic disorders requires special skills and a great deal of sensitivity and understanding. The ophthalmic nurse must keep abreast of recent advances in both nursing practice and technological development, and this third edition of *Ophthalmic Nursing* is written with this in mind.

The text is written for all nurses who will care for ophthalmic patients, whether as part of their general nurse training or at a post-basic level.

We have stressed throughout the importance of individualized patient care using a problem-solving approach. More detail has been given on key points of nursing care for specific ophthalmic conditions and on dealing with patients as people. New chapters have been included on theatre and out-patient nursing, traumatic injury, the eye and general health, and services available to the visually handicapped.

We hope that the book will provide the basic information needed to carry out sensitive nursing care and that it will provide a stimulus to nurses to explore ophthalmic nursing more fully.

March 1987   MARY KIRTON
                                               MARY RICHARDSON

Acknowledgements

Our special thanks are due to the following people:

Brigid Knight, tutor at the Wolfson School of Nursing, Westminster Hospital, for contributing the first and last chapters.

Rosemary Morris, Nursing Editor at Baillière Tindall, for all her help and encouragement with the project.

Dr Tom Barrie, Consultant Ophthalmologist at Glasgow Eye Infirmary, and Katie Booth, who read the text and made many helpful comments.

Ian Smith, who took the new photographs , and Ian Kirton, who posed for many of them.

Miss Blair, Senior Nurse at Gartnaval General Hospital, for her help and cooperation.

Carrie Bennet and Katy Macauley for their very efficient typing.

Our long-suffering and understanding loved ones, especially Claire, aged two, who obligingly went to bed so it could all be written.

1 Introduction

by Brigid Knight

Man now lives in a relatively safe world and the need to possess very acute senses of touch, taste, hearing and smell in order to survive has decreased. He relies very much on his sight to inform him of impending pleasure or danger, so if anything occurs to decrease or destroy his vision, it alters the efficiency of his inter-action with the environment in which he lives.

The search to find ways of correcting visual handicap is a long established one, couching of cataracts having been recorded in 2000 BC: this simply meant exerting pressure on the eye, causing the opaque lens to dislocate and drop out of the light pathway into the vitreous chamber, and after transient restoration of some degree of sight, often resulted in a painful, irreversible blindness. Despite this fact, it was really the only operation being performed until the first iridotomy by Cheselden in the 1730s and the first planned cataract extraction by Daviel in 1742.

As long ago as 1847, Sir William Bowman, a surgeon at Moor-fields (then the Royal London Ophthalmic Hospital) recognized the importance of those caring for his patients being trained to do so. He established St John's House, the nurses from which were given lectures by doctors from King's College Hospital. The Order of St John took over the actual running of the hospital in 1856 to establish control over the quality of care given, and to improve it. In 1952 the Ophthalmic Nursing Board came into being, so setting a national standard for pre- and post-basic courses and examinations. They are due to come under the aus-pices of the English National Board in 1988.

The role of the ophthalmic nurse is multi-facetted in that she assists in the prevention of visual handicap, in the restoration of sight, and if necessary, in the adaptation of the individual to any degree of alteration in his vision.

Prevention requires the acquisition of knowledge and a continu-ing interest in current trends, thinking and research in order to give up-to-date information to her patients.

An awareness of potentially damaging practices such as working without protective goggles, or inadequate cleaning of contact lenses may prevent many ophthalmic problems if this information is used as a health education resource.

Some conditions are familial, and the identification of those at risk, plus the organization of systematic follow-up will result in early diagnosis or prevention of potentially crippling visual conditions such as glaucoma or strabismus.

Most of the ophthalmic nurse's time is spent in caring for the person who is being treated medically and/or surgically for a condition that threatens his visual acuity to a varying degree. This requires certain skills and aptitudes, and the acceptance that the pace and atmosphere of an ophthalmic unit is different from many other clinical areas, as the needs of the patients are very different. It is not easy or ideal to nurse ophthalmic patients on general surgical wards, as it often results in their needs being negated in the general day-to-day hurly burly.

Patients admitted for ophthalmic treatment are often faced with the possibility of losing their sight, because although the aim of all treatment is to maintain or, if at all possible, improve their visual acuity, there is always the possibility that something may go wrong. This underlying, sometimes irrational fear may result in displays of anger, aggression or withdrawal on the part of the patient: the nurse must realize this and respond appropriately.

Good communication is the key; the ability to establish quickly a trusting relationship with, and instil confidence in the patient is all-important from the very beginning: there is a need to be empathic without being condescending, and to have an awareness that many of the elements of non-verbal communication will not be appreciated by someone who is visually handicapped.

The importance of touch as a substitute for non-verbal reinforcement cannot be stressed enough, but this will depend on the individual. The nurse will also have to accept being touched, as someone with a profound handicap will often say that they do not 'know' someone until they have touched his or her face, and perhaps hands. Contact with another person at a time of stress can be very therapeutic.

A sighted person will often interpret what they hear in combination with the expression on the speaker's face, as the latter can add to, or detract from, what is being said. The blind or partially sighted person cannot always do this, so tone of voice takes on a much greater meaning, and the nurse should appreciate the possibility of being misinterpreted at times. This factor can be compounded by the heightening of other senses as one deteriorates, and those whose sight has worsened often say that their hearing has become more acute; their sensory input alters and this can be confusing, not to say frightening. This fear can be greatly decreased by making sure that all extraneous noises are kept to a minimum, and a full explanation of all noises is given—the person in question cannot see what is coming towards them, and even the tea trolley can become an object of fear!

The timing and frequency of communication must be considered carefully: anxiety, advanced age and insecurity make the rapid assimilation of information very difficult for the individual. It should not be assumed that someone else has given the patient information, especially if there is the slightest chance that it was given at the same time as the patient was told that he would need surgery or that their vision would continue to deteriorate—anxiety blocks understanding very effectively. All opportunities need to be used to convey new information, consolidate that given previously and answer any queries that arise. It may require great patience on the nurse's part as the same queries are often repeated again and again, and despite repeated reassurance and explanation, the patient may continue to demonstrate lack of understanding by his behaviour.

Adaptability is an essential quality required when caring for the visually handicapped because, apart from anything else, the age of patients may vary from birth to over 100, although children should ideally be nursed in a paediatric unit. This diversity in age can necessitate the acquisition of a wide range of talents, from mending toys, telling stories and retrieving dropped knitting stitches to taking part in a discussion about fashions in the 1890s with a lady who had been the assistant to Queen Victoria's mantua-maker—you learn an awful lot about all sorts of things.

This situation can be relieved by being aware of and being prepared to use the resources available: older patients will often happily sit and read stories to the youngest ones; and many old men, and not so old, return to childhood at the sight of a train set. This sometimes requires the application of tact and diplomacy because, if the activity is detrimental to the patient's condition, it is often demonstrated that 70- and 80-year-olds can sulk! Activities such as the construction of the railway line between the cubicle and bed nine may well ease the transportation of supplies from an adopted 'grandad' to the child, but can be an obstacle to other patients, and so ingenuity is required to veto or tactfully re-route this engineering project.

However, many of the patients in ophthalmic units are elderly but, despite their age, may have never been in hospital, and so can be confused by a new place, different routine and ignorance of what is expected of them. Many who have been in before will have been in for the treatment of a childhood ailment, at a time when hospital routine was much more strictly regimented and they are often afraid of doing something wrong.

They may also find that, although they have been coping with the day-to-day activities at home, bringing them out of a familiar environment makes them more dependent and can increase the anxiety they may already be feeling: this can lead to mental confusion, a situation that needs careful handling and explanation, not only for the patient, but also for family and friends.

All concerned will be aware that the success or failure of the treatment may well determine the patients' dependence on, or independence of, others, and in some cases may be the factor that decides whether the individual stays at home or goes to live with the family or in sheltered accommodation.

The nurse needs sensitivity to recognize and take measures to alleviate, as far as possible, the anxieties being felt, but there may be other elements to consider.

The individual with a visual handicap such as cataracts, which is often seen as a temporary problem existing only until they are ready for surgery, will probably have had little in the way of formal help to adjust to his failing sight, and may have coped by retreating into the home and only leaving to go to familar surroundings, leading to isolation and the loss of social skills. This problem will be compounded by any degree of anxiety, and it requires understanding and skilful persuasion to help the patient integrate into the social unit of the ward. The problem may be as basic as a fear of being thought 'messy' at mealtimes, causing the patient to refuse to sit at the table with others, lest they spill food due to their inability to see the plate properly: simple aids such as plate guards and non-slip mats may help.

One of the great bonuses of ophthalmic nursing is to see some-one who, on admission, is withdrawn and frightened blossom into an interesting, independent being. It is part of the nurse's responsibility to see that, after this metamorphosis, the patient does not return to isolation on discharge, a situation that he may find intolerably depressing. This is especially true if, although their sight has been improved, they are on their own or have a degree of physical handicap, because immobility or a fear of going out on their own may prevent them from socializing: referral to the Social Services with a view to attendance at a Day Centre or Luncheon Club may overcome this.

Some people are more perceptive than others, and the development and understanding of perception are skills that the ophthalmic nurse should cultivate.

Perception is the process by which we organize and interpret the patterns of stimuli in our environment; how we make sense of what we sense. An individual's perception is altered by past experience and present needs. This applies not only to the patient but also to the nurse: we are all less perceptive at times; pressure at work and state of mind can all affect the way we interpret things. Vision plays a major part in perception; by allowing the appreciation of colour, shading and change in form the three-dimensional world becomes apparent, and the appreciation of movement and change provides a sense of time.

No two individuals with normal vision and a settled state of mind will perceive a situation identically, so it must be realized that someone with a visual handicap and a potentially high anxiety level may have a very different perception of the situation altogether from others who are in the same position.

Visual handicap can vary in its intensity, presentation and permanence: it may be the family rather than the individual who first notice that the normally spotless house has cobwebs and a layer of dust or that the person's clothes are stained and dirty, a situation that would normally be unacceptable for that person. This in itself requires very tactful handling by the family, and may need the conciliatory skills of the nurse in the out-patients department.

The patient may complain of the loss of colour appreciation and lack of detail, especially if they are developing cataracts. Painters such as Turner have style changes attributed to cataract development: the clear primary colours and detail of his Venetian painting give way to the less detailed, duller representation of

'The Thames at Walton Bridge' and to the rather obscure red/
brown/yellow swirl of the 'Fighting Temeraire'.

Diseases such as glaucoma cause a constriction of the visual field
and it may be a 'near miss' collision with someone or something
approaching from the side that causes the individual to realize
that he has a diminished peripheral field of vision.

Gradual deterioration in vision allows the affected person time
to adjust and prepare, especially if the cause is untreatable: it is
the sudden loss of vision due to an accident, for instance, that is
probably harder to cope with.

Many of the skills needed to help someone adjust to an alteration in their level of visual acuity are the same as those required
to care for someone having restorative ocular surgery. The major
difference in many cases is that little or no hope can be offered
to the individual, and the ultimate goal must be to instil in them
a feeling of optimism about the future and what it holds.

It is difficult to imagine what it is like to be irreversibly blind
or partially sighted. We can close our eyes and appreciate the
physical problems but we know that, when we open them, we
will see—the psychological fear and despair are not there. Every
day we take for granted the range of colour and images that come
before us, and it is not until vision starts to fail that the enormity
of it all becomes apparent. Nurses need to realize this when
working with the visually handicapped; they are the eyes of the
patients and need imagination to describe form and colours accurately. The family can play a considerable part in this, as they
can relate the present to the past, and draw on the patient's
previous knowledge and experience to bring the world to life
again.

Much will depend on the individual's expectations: an old lady
whose main pleasure in living is sitting down listening to the radio
may not find the prospect of losing her vision as distressing as a
young man for whom the loss of sight may necessitate a change
of job, role within the family and lifestyle.

Reactions will vary from acceptance and a dogged determi-
nation to overcome the handicap to a deep reactionary depression
that requires psychiatric help. The nurse must have the ability to
respond to any coping mechanism the patient devises and
employs: to encourage when small realistic goals are set and
attained, and to sympathize when they are not, but to offer

constructive suggestions as to how they could be. The nurse's listening skills are all important; the patient may be reluctant to express his fears and feelings to his family and friends initially, and so time must be allowed for this.

These fears may express themselves in outbursts of anger and self pity, and it is important for the establishment of an effective trusting relationship that the nurse recognizes them for what they are. The outbursts may come after the failure to achieve something, and the temptation that the nurse faces is to step in and do it. Although this may initially make life easier, it increases the individual's dependence on others in the long term. To stand and watch is probably one of the most difficult things a nurse has to learn to do, but it is infinitely more difficult for the family, because patients will often employ a strategy that can only be described as emotional blackmail when trying to get them to do something for them. All concerned need a great deal of help and understanding at this time.

The nurse's primary role is to maintain a safe environment in which the visually handicapped person can gain confidence and learn by trial and error, but the nurse should only intervene to offer constructive help or to prevent physical injury. The patient should be informed of any unusual obstacles, and the position of furniture, equipment and personal belongings should remain constant, as apart from causing physical harm, confidence lost after a fall takes a long time to be re-established. The relationship between the nurse, the patient and the family is very important, and can be one of the most satisfying aspects of ophthalmic nursing: fears of a fundamental change in a way of life or role on behalf of the patient, and consequently the partner, may mean that a relationship is established at a deeper level than in many other branches of nursing. All parties need explanation of one another's fears and feelings, and to be encouraged to express them to one another. The nurse must take on the role of a facilitator and information source, and although accepting negative thoughts, must put forward a positive viewpoint and display confidence in order to give all concerned the strength to continue.

It is often difficult for someone who is struggling to re-establish themselves as a useful member of society in their own eyes to laugh at themselves: but a sense of humour is so important on all sides, and the nurse should always be ready to laugh with her patients when appropriate. Laughter can make yet another failure to achieve a goal a little less daunting, but it must always be perfectly clear to the patient what the laughter is about: their inability to identify the cause of amusement may increase their feeling of social isolation.

It can also help if they learn to laugh at the activities of those trying to help them; as in the case of the gentleman who, on reaching the out-patients department unaccompanied by his wife for the first time since losing his sight, vowed never to stop to get his bearings again. Each time he had, some kind member of the public had taken him across the road! He had also seen the amusing side of it, and had thanked each person, because he realized that an angry response might mean that they would be reluctant to help others in future.

It also needs to be accepted that the restoration of vision can be frightening: an artist, Edward Ardizzone, said that having his cataracts removed introduced him to a 'colder, brighter world' and he missed 'the smaller, kind, rather misty world' he had loved so well. Some people cope by still not seeing although there is no physical reason why they should not do so. Seeing again can also be quite depressing, for they can suddenly see with awful clarity how much they and their families have aged!

The primary colours especially can take on a frightening intensity; they seem unreal and are difficult to comprehend and accept unless there is an understanding of the changes that have taken place. Decreased visual acuity has often been used an as excuse for not doing things, and suddenly the excuse has been removed: the individual, family and friends may need to look beyond the handicap to the real cause of their reluctance to do things.

Nursing ophthalmic patients requires a great deal of understanding, sensitivity and patience, but also the awareness of the need to keep in touch with other aspects of nursing. Many patients will have other medical conditions; some directly related to the visual handicap, others due to their age. As mentioned before, it is often the first time that the person has been in hospital and a thorough pre-operative assessment may identify previously unknown medical conditions, and it may be the nurse who has to explain the condition, investigations and treatment required. Provided that the nurse is prepared to accept the differences between working with ophthalmic patients and some others, that the work may be less physically trying but calls for a greater degree of emotional involvement, the advantages are numerous.

Whatever the outcome of treatment, the satisfaction of seeing someone return to his proper place in society is considerable.

There can be little more satisfying than seeing the joy, relief and sometimes tears on the face of someone who has had surgery and who, although his vision when the dressing is removed may be far from perfect, can appreciate the light and colour that have been missed for so long.

The results may not always be so dramatic, but just as satisfying. Amy Cameron's vision had been poor all her life; now she was blind. She had sought no treatment, because when she was younger she had been told there was nothing that could help: now, in her seventies, her family had persuaded her to see an ophthalmologist because of advances that had been made in this field of medicine. The consultant had made no promises, but three days before Amy had undergone a combined cataract extraction/ corneal graft with little immediate improvement. On the day in question, the Queen was coming to open a new department in the hospital and Amy desperately wanted to go down to the front hall and 'feel' the atmosphere. She was wheeled down to a front row seat, but on her return was so excited: 'The Queen was wearing a beautiful turquoise coat. I could see it!'

For everyone in the ward that evening, the topic of conversation was not only the Queen's visit.

FURTHER READING

Frisby, J.P. (1979) *Seeing Illusion, Brain and Mind.* Oxford: Oxford University Press.
Gregory, R.L. (1977) *Eye and Brian: The Psychology of Seeing,* London: Weidenfeld & Nicolson.
Hilgard, E.R., Atkinson, R.L. & Atkinson, R.C. (1979) '*An Introduction to Psychology.* New York: Harcourt Brace Jovanovich.
Trevor-Roper, P.D. (1970) *The World Through Blunted Sight.* London: Thames & Hudson.

2 The eye

The eyeball measures almost 25 mm in diameter and is surrounded by pads of fat within the bony orbit. It is unprotected only on its anterior surface where the cornea lies. The cornea is more convex than the rest of the eyeball, so that there is an anterior prominence in an otherwise almost complete sphere (see Fig. 2.1).

The three lining layers of the eye, the sclera, the choroid and the retina, enclose the transparent media of aqueous humour, lens and vitreous humour.

THE OUTER SHELL

The *sclera* covers the posterior five-sixths of the eyeball and is composed of interlaced bands of tough, fibrous tissue with a poor blood supply. Although known as the 'white of the eye' its colour

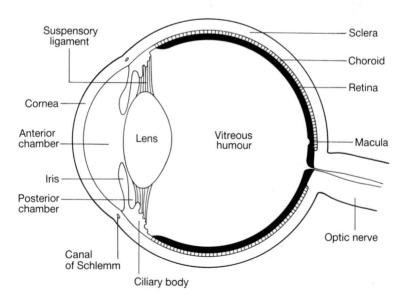

Fig. 2.1 *Section through the eyeball to show the major structures.*

varies from bluish in children to yellowish in the elderly. The *cornea* is continuous with the sclera and covers the anterior portion of the eye. It is transparent and avascular and sensory nerve endings within it respond only to pain.

THE UVEAL TRACT

The *choroid*, the middle lining layer, is vascular and pigmented, appearing dark brown in colour. It is responsible for the blood supply to the outer layers of the retina.

The *ciliary body* forms a ring connecting the choroid with the iris; it is black and triangular in section. Aqueous is produced in the ciliary processes, a series of about 70 ridges surrounding the lens margin. The ciliary muscle fibres connect the sclera with the ciliary processes and are used to alter the convexity of the lens in the process of accommodation.

The *iris* is the anterior part of the middle layer of the coats of the eye and is a disc perforated at its centre by the pupil. The colour of the iris depends on the amount of pigment it contains. Smooth muscle fibres within the iris are responsible for constricting and dilating the pupil.

THE RETINA

The transparent *retina* contains many nerve fibres and receptors and is the innermost layer of the eye. It leaves the eye at the *optic nerve* and has a small depression at its posterior pole the *macula lutea*. In the centre of the macula is the *fovea centralis*, the area responsible for detailed vision. Two types of photoreceptor are found in the retina. *Rods* contain the pigment rhodopsin or visual purple and allow vision in poor illumination. There are no rods in the fovea but their numbers increase towards the periphery of the retina. *Cones* are present in large numbers at the fovea, with fewer elsewhere in the retina. They are concerned with detailed vision in conditions of bright illumination and also colour vision; three photochemical pigments in the cones are broken down by light of different ranges of wavelengths and provide the sensations of red, green and blue colours.

INTERNAL STRUCTURES

Aqueous humour is a colourless fluid that is actively secreted from cells lining the ciliary body into the *posterior chamber*. It circulates through the pupil into the *anterior chamber* and nourishes the lens and its capsule, the suspensory ligament and the cornea. Aqueous is formed at a rate of about 0.5 ml per day and maintains the intra-ocular pressure at 15–20 mmHg. It drains via the *canal of Schlemm* (Fig. 2.1).

The transparent, biconvex body of *the lens* is situated between the iris and the vitreous body and is held in position by *suspensory ligaments*. It is the focusing mechanism of the eye: it has different curvatures at the centre and periphery of its anterior surface so that light is bent at different angles and is focused at the fovea.

Vitreous humour is a semi-fluid, transparent, gelatinous substance which fills the *vitreous body* and does not regenerate.

The *extra-ocular muscles* are concerned with moving the eye in all directions, the two eyes being coordinated in normal vision. The four recti muscles and the two oblique muscles are illustrated in Fig. 2.2.

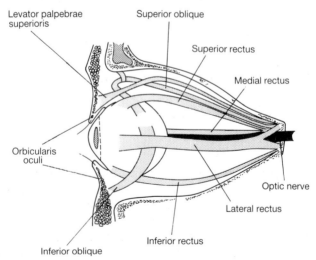

Fig. 2.2 *The muscles of the eye. The eye is moved by small muscles which link the sclera to the bony orbit. Acting together, the extrinsic muscles can bring about rotatory movement. Both eyes normally move together so that images fall on corresponding points of both retinae.*

NERVE AND BLOOD SUPPLY

Sensory nerve supply is from branches of the trigeminal nerve (Vth cranial). Motor nerves are supplied by both sympathetic (responsible for pupil dilation and for blood flow) and parasympathetic (pupillary constriction) systems. The *optic nerve* (IInd cranial) enters the orbit via the foramen, and runs forwards and slightly outwards and downwards (to allow for eye movements) before attaching to the back of the eye. As the nerve enters the eye, the fibres lose their myelin sheath and pass through the sclera and choroid to become continuous with the nerve layer of the retina at the *optic disc*. The optic nerve contains about one million individual fibres.

Blood supply to the eyeball and orbital contents is mainly from the ophthalmic artery, with the eyelids and conjunctiva being additionally supplied by branches of the external carotid artery. The ophthalmic artery, a branch of the internal carotid, enters the orbit through the foramen below and lateral to the optic nerve before subdividing to supply the various parts of the eye. Venous drainage is mainly through the superior and inferior orbital veins which are tortuous, valveless and empty into the cavernous sinus.

THE VISUAL PATHWAY

In order to know what we are looking at, we need:

> Light
> A functioning eye
> Refractive media
> Photoreceptors

Light passes through the clear refractive media (cornea, aqueous, lens and vitreous) and is brought to a focus on the fovea because it is bent at the various refracting surfaces of the eye, notably at the cornea and the anterior surface of the lens. When rods and cones are stimulated by light their photochemical pigments are broken down; this action sets off a nerve impulse which is transmitted via the optic nerve to the visual centres in the occipital cortex. The optic nerves from both eyes join at the optic chiasma and the nasal fibres from each eye cross over to the opposite side

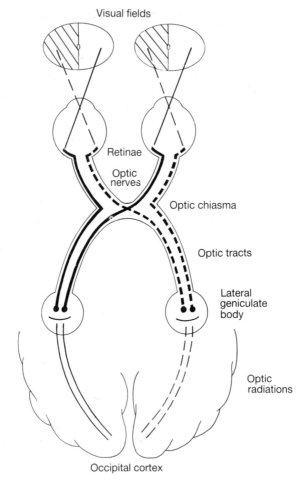

Fig. 2.3 *The visual pathways.*

(decussate) (see Fig. 2.3). The left half of the visual field is thus seen by the right half of the brain, and vice versa. The visual cortex receives two slightly different images of the same object and fuses them to form a single three-dimensional mental impression.

FURTHER READING

Wolff, E. (1976) *Anatomy of the Eye and Orbit*, 7th Edn. London: H.K. Lewis.

3 Examination of the eye

When a patient presents at the out-patient department with an injured or diseased eye, careful examination of the eye must be undertaken and visual acuity established in order that future improvement or deterioration may be accurately assessed. An individualized approach is important if the full implications of the patient's ophthalmic problems are to be seen in the context of his or her daily life. What may be a serious problem for one patient may cause only minor inconvenience to another because of the different nature of the normal daily routine.

Ophthalmic history will help to determine any long-standing or familial problems. The patient should be asked about his general health including current medications and any known allergies. If headaches are experienced, the location, duration and intensity of the pain should be noted, as should anything that relieves or exacerbates the pain. Patients whose vision is already corrected, whether myopic or hypermetropic, should be asked whether their spectacles or lenses relieve any symptoms. Double vision in any direction should be detected, and any history of eye discharge, clear or purulent, should be recorded. When a patient presents with an eye injury, it is vital to obtain a history of what he was doing and using at the time.

While questioning her patient, the nurse must observe him carefully. If a ptosis, proptosis or squint is present, she should note this. The patient may tilt his head in order to overcome diplopia.

OBJECTIVE EXAMINATION OF THE EYE

The patient should be seated in a comfortable chair with a head-rest, and the nurse should explain the examination procedure to him, reassuring him that he will not feel any pain. The face should be observed for rosacea, which may affect the eyelids, and for any evidence of discharge from the eyes.

Bruising and swelling of the skin around the orbits should be noted, as should the position of the eyes within the orbits and any displacement of the eyeballs. Eyelids should not be crusted or ulcerated and any abnormality of the eyelashes will be evident on close examination. Any swelling of the lacrimal sac area or poor drainage of tears through the lacrimal puncta should be recorded. To examine the conjunctiva properly it will be necessary to evert the upper eyelid (see Fig. 3.1); any foreign bodies, injection, dryness or scarring will then be readily seen. The cornea should be examined for infiltrations, opacities, inflammation and corneal foreign bodies; corneal abrasions or ulceration will show up as a bright green stain if a drop of Gutt. Fluorescein 2% is instilled into the eye and washed out with isotonic saline. The depth of the anterior chamber should be observed, as should the presence of blood or pus in the normally clear aqueous humour. The nurse should note the colour of the irides while looking for any signs of thickening or swelling and noting any missing parts, as in a coloboma or following iridectomy. Adhesions of the iris, trembling of the iris when the eye is moved (iridodonesis) and

Place little finger at rim   Draw upper lid down
of tarsal plate   and slightly out

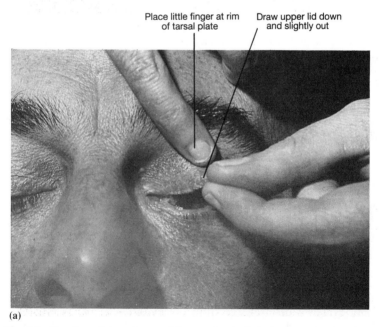

(a)

Fig. 3.1 *Everting of the upper eyelid using (a) the little finger, and (b) a glass rod. (c) The upper eyelid everted.*

Place glass rod at rim of tarsal plate   Draw upper lid down and slightly out

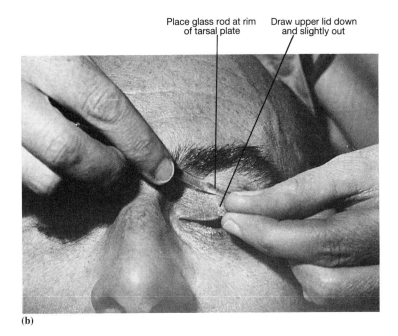

(b)

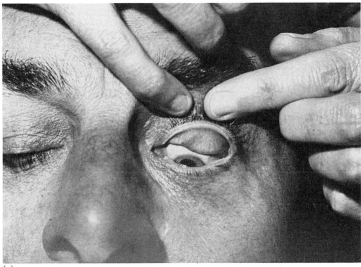

(c)

tearing of the iris away from its root (iridodialysis) should be excluded. The pupils should be examined in order to detect any abnormality in size or shape and to ensure that no membrane is present. Their reaction to light may be tested using a hand torch—it is important that the nurse explains the procedure to the patient in order to gain his co-operation. Any pigmentation or cataract in the lens can be seen by direct vision, as may be subluxation or dislocations of the lens.

The patient should be asked to close his eyes and look down so that the nurse may gently palpate over his upper eyelids (see Fig. 3.2) in order to detect any orbital swelling or grossly raised intra-ocular pressure. The patient may complain of discomfort over any area of episcleritis. Intra-ocular pressure may then be measured with a tonometer (Fig. 3.3).

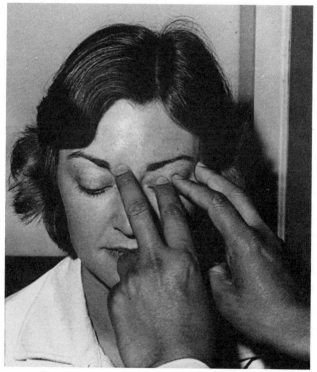

Fig. 3.2 *Testing the tension of the eyeball laterally.*

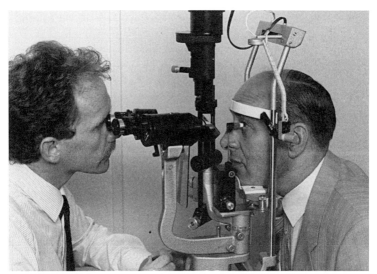

Fig. 3.3 *Applanation tonometry. The patient must keep his chin on the rest and his forehead at the band when the tonometer is applied to the cornea.*

Whenever possible, the nurse should take the opportunity of examining the posterior part of the eyeball with the direct and indirect ophthalmoscope under the guidance of an ophthalmologist. In order to facilitate this procedure, the patient's pupils may be dilated with a mydriatic such as cyclopentolate. The action may later be reversed by a miotic, or the patient may be detained until the effect of the eye drops has partly worn off.

Through the ophthalmoscope (Fig. 3.4) the doctor will look for any abnormality in the vitreous such as haemorrhage or fibrous bands. The retinal blood vessels will be examined and any abnormalities in the macula area will be excluded. The optic disc will be viewed so that any swelling, cupping or other abnormality can be noted. The entire retina will then be examined for abnormalities; it will be necessary to use an indirect ophthalmoscope to view the periphery.

VISUAL ACUITY

Visual acuity is the facility the eye possesses of perceiving the shape or form of objects from a distance. Normal development

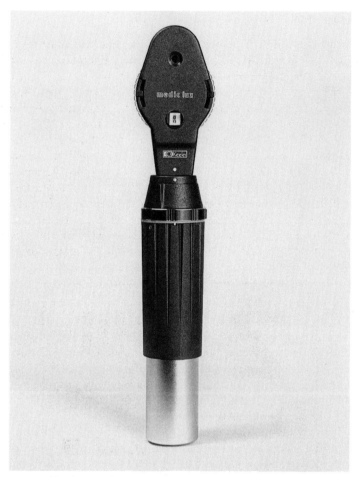

Fig. 3.4 *A direct ophthalmoscope. By courtesy of Keeler.*

of visual acuity requires not only normal anatomical structure but also normal visual experience for reinforcement. Visual functions develop rapidly in the early years of life and are acutely sensitive in the first two or three years. For proper binocular co-ordination, the individual needs good, and preferably equal, visual acuity in each eye. Testing visual acuity is an essential part of the examination of the eye. It is normally done by the nurse, who needs to be familiar with the various testing methods available for both distant and near vision.

Distant vision

Distant vision is tested using a well illuminated test chart set at a distance of 6 m from the patient. If space is limited a chart with reversed test type can be reflected in a mirror set at 3 m from the patient. The charts consist of a series of letters graduated in size and arranged in horizontal rows. The large top letter can normally be read at 60 m and the subsequent rows at 36, 24, 18, 12, 9 and 6 m. A person with normal vision will be able to read the smallest type at 6 m and his visual acuity would be recorded as 6/6. Someone who could read only the large, top letter would have a visual acuity of 6/60. The upper figure, the numerator, is the distance in metres from the chart—usually 6 m. The lower figure, or denominator, refers to the size of the smallest letters that the patient can read accurately. The most commonly used chart is Snellen's Test Type (see Fig. 3.5). The 'E' type chart can

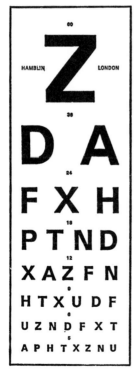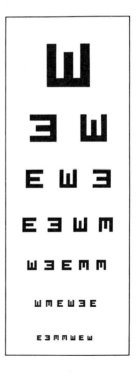

Fig. 3.5 *(a) Snellen's test types. (b) 'E' test types.*

be used with pre-school children or illiterate adults. The client is given a large E and asked to turn it in the same direction as the various E's on the chart (Fig. 3.5). The Bealle Collins and Kay Tests have graded pictures and are useful with those under three years old (Fig. 3.6). The Sheridan Gardiner Test is also useful with young children: the nurse shows a book or block with one letter on each page or side, graded in size, and the child is asked to point to the correct letter on a card which he holds (Fig. 3.7). Coloured balls or sweets can be used with babies or very small children.

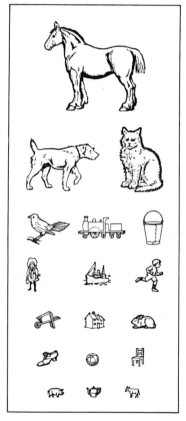

Fig. 3.6 *(a) 'B1474' test types. (b) Kay test:* **left**, *chart to ensure that the patient can identify the pictures;* **upper right**, *book with pictures for the patient to hold;* **lower right**, *book with pictures in graded sizes that the nurse holds.*

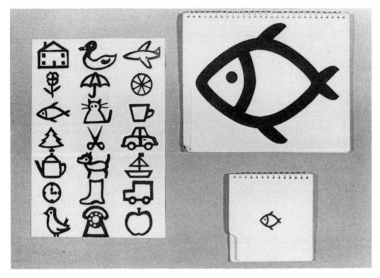

Fig. 3.6 *(b)*

The patient should have one eye tested at a time, with the other properly but lightly occluded. Pressing the palm of the hand on the occluded eye will cause distortion of vision in that eye. Time must be allowed for the 'second' eye to adapt to light. Those

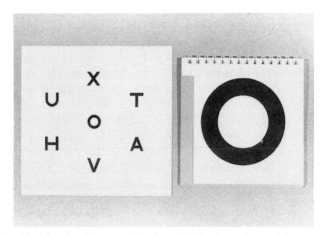

Fig. 3.7 *Sheridan Gardiner test.* **Left** *chart held by the patient and letter pointed to when identified.* **Right** *book held by nurse with one letter per page in graded sizes.*

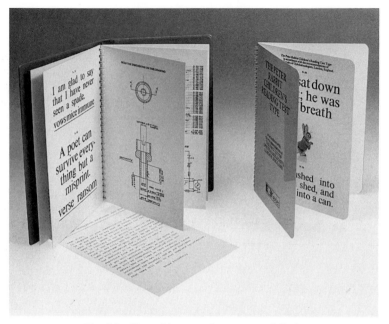

Fig. 3.8 *Near vision test. By courtesy of Keeler.*

patients who wear glasses for distant vision should wear these glasses when having their visual acuity tested.

If the patient is unable to read the large letter at 6 m, he is moved forward a metre at a time until he can read it. The numerator will then be the distance in metres from the board, e.g. 2/60. A patient who cannot see the large letter at 1 m will be asked to count the tester's fingers at 0.5 m (recorded as CF); if he is unable to do this he may be able to see hand movements (HM). Some patients are unable to perceive hand movements but can perceive light. A torch is shone into their eyes from different directions. If the patient can tell the direction from which the light is coming, this is recorded as accurate projection of light; if he can see the light but not the direction, 'perception of light' is recorded. In a few instances there may be no perception of light.

Most test type charts can be changed to eliminate the possibility of patients, particularly those who frequently attend an ophthalmic clinic, memorizing the letters.

Near vision

Near vision is tested by asking the patient to read from a card containing paragraphs with different letter sizes. The card should be well lit and held at the normal reading distance from the eye, 33 cm. The N series of test types or Jaeger's test type are generally used (Fig. 3.8). Patients who wear glasses for reading should be tested wearing their reading glasses.

Visual field tests

Visual field tests aim to define the area of vision in an eye during an undeviated, straight-ahead gaze. A number of ophthalmic diseases cause a reduction, either central or peripheral, in the visual field. The central visual field is 'picked up' almost exclusively by the cones which are densest at the macula, while light from the peripheral field falls almost exclusively on the rods of the retina. There is inevitably a blind spot over the optic disc but any other area of blindness in the visual field is referred to as a *scotoma*.

The Confrontation Test can be used to identify gross visual field defects. The patient is asked to sit facing the tester and at arm's length from him, and to cover the left eye lightly with his hand. He then looks with his right eye at the examiner's left eye while the examiner slowly brings his fingers into the patient's line of sight. The patient is asked to indicate as soon as he can see the fingers. The test is repeated at 30–45 degree intervals around the 360 degree periphery for each eye. The fullness of the reported field is compared to that of the tester. Both peripheral and central fields are then more accurately recorded using an analyser (Fig. 3.9), a Bjerrum screen test and an Amsler recording chart (Fig. 3.10). The Amsler chart records macular function.

Colour vision tests

Colour vision defects (often incorrectly called 'colour blindness') may be either acquired or hereditary. Hereditary defects occur in 8% of the male and 0.5% of the female population and most commonly result in inability to distinguish between red and green.

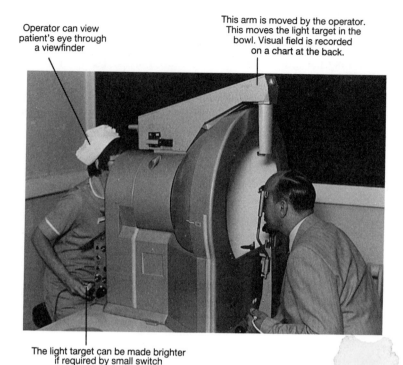

Operator can view patient's eye through a viewfinder

This arm is moved by the operator. This moves the light target in the bowl. Visual field is recorded on a chart at the back.

The light target can be made brighter if required by small switch

Fig. 3.9 *The Tubinger Analyser, Central and peripheral visual fields are recorded with this machine.*

This may be a problem in some industries in which colour differentiation is important, or in driving, navigating or piloting when incorrect interpretation of a coloured light or signal may have drastic consequences.

The Ishihara Test (Fig. 3.11) only tests for red/green defects. A number formed of coloured dots is surrounded by a background in another colour. Only those with normal colour vision can see the number. The Farnsworth–Munsell 100 Hue Test is a more complex test and is particularly useful for detecting acquired colour vision defects. The patient is asked to arrange 85 different colours according to hue, sometimes with a time limit of five minutes. Each eye is tested separately, and the number of errors made within each of four hue groups will indicate the type and severity of the colour vision defect.

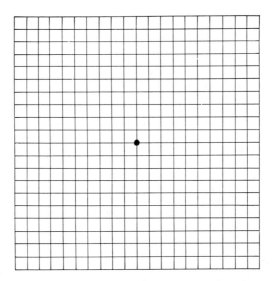

Fig. 3.10 *The Amsler recording chart. The patient is asked to hold this chart and concentrate on the central spot. If macular function is impaired, the small squares will be distorted.*

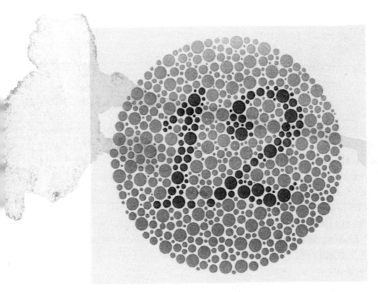

Fig. 3.11 *Ishihara Colour Vision Test. This is a plate composed of coloured circles. A number, which the patient must identify, is formed in circles of one colour.*

TREATMENTS AND TECHNIQUES

Before undertaking any of the procedures outlined below, the nurse should ensure that she is fully aware of, and adheres to, the local policy regarding the extended role of the nurse. Further, it is her responsibility to ensure that she is competent at such procedures before attempting to perform them unsupervised.

Many patients will be fearful of the thought of treatment to their eyes and it is essential for the nurse to gain their confidence and co-operation. A full explanation must be given to the patient using terms that he can understand; this should include warning him if the procedure may be uncomfortable or painful. He should be seated or lying comfortably with his head well supported, so that he is as relaxed as possible.

Bathing the eye is a simple procedure but must be carried out with great care. Each eye should be treated separately, with the nurse ensuring that her hands are thoroughly cleaned before treating each eye. She should always work from the side of the eye being bathed. Requirements include:

> Torch
> Sterile gallipot
> Sterile wool balls
> Sterile towel
> Isotonic saline
> Disposal bag

The nurse should drape the patient with the sterile towel and ask him to close his eye. Bathing is done with a saline-moistened sterile swab drawn gently along the eyelid margins from the inner canthus outwards. Each swab should be used only once and then discarded. Bathing should continue until the eyelids are clean; the lower eyelid may be drawn down slightly while the patient looks up so that crusts may be removed from the lower lid and lashes. The skin should be dried with a cotton wool swab once bathing is complete. Check that the eyelids are clean with the aid of a torch.

It is important not to exert undue pressure on the eyeball and not to touch the eyeball, particularly the cornea. If a patient has sustained an intra-ocular injury or undergone intra-ocular surgery, the top of the upper eyelid should not be swabbed unless absolutely necessary.

Everting the upper lid is carried out as follows. The patient is asked to look down while the nurse, standing behind him, holds his lashes between her thumb and forefinger. The lid is drawn down and out from the eyeball, and is turned back over a glass rod or the little finger of the nurse's other hand, which is used to depress the upper edge of the tarsal plate (Fig. 3.12). The lid may be kept everted while rodding or irrigation are carried out.

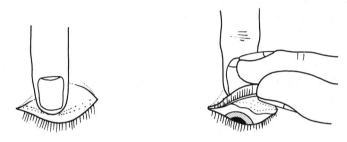

Fig. 3.12 *Eversion of the upper eyelid.*

Irrigating the eye is most commonly carried out following chemical splashes, either acid or alkaline, to the eye. Requirements include:

> Irrigating solution at the correct temperature
> Giving set or container (squeezy bottle, 20 ml syringe or undine) for solution
> Receiver for returned solution, e.g. a kidney dish
> Gutt. Benoxinate 0.4% or Gutt. Amethocaine 1%
> Glass rod
> Protection for patient's clothing

The patient must be lying with his head on one pillow or seated in a reclined chair with a headrest. His clothing should be protected and he should be asked to tilt his head to the affected side and to hold the receiver in a suitable position to collect the return wash. An anaesthetic drop such as Gutt. Benoxinate 0.4% may be instilled to make the procedure more comfortable. The nurse should stand behind the patient, ask him to look up, and gently

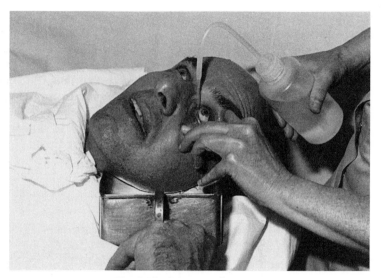

Fig. 3.13 *Irrigation of an eye.*

draw down the lower eyelid. She should allow some of the irrigation solution to run over the patient's cheek (Fig. 3.13) to
ensure that it is at a suitable temperature, and so that he knows
when to expect the fluid in his eye. The lower fornix should then
be irrigated from the medial canthus outwards. The upper fornix
is irrigated by drawing up the upper lid and asking the patient to
look down. The upper lid should then be everted (a glass rod
may be required) and irrigation continued. Effective irrigation
takes at least 20 minutes and should be continued until the pH
of the patient's tears returns to within normal limits. The fornices
must be carefully examined at the end of the procedure and the
patient should be left dry and comfortable. The cornea may then
be stained with Gutt. Fluorescein 2% to exclude any corneal
abrasions.

Instilling drops and ointments requires great care on the part of
the nurse to ensure that the eye is not damaged or infected.
Requirements are as for bathing the eye plus:

> Appropriate eye drops or ointments
> Patient prescription sheet

The eye is bathed first to ensure that it is clean and free from previous medication. The nurse should work from the side of the affected eye so that at no time is medication passed across the unaffected side. Eye drops or ointments are checked against the patient's prescription and only those appropriate to the eye being treated should be opened. If multi-dose preparations are used, care must be taken to ensure that the screw top is kept clean, preferably by placing it on a sterile towel. The patient is asked to look upwards, his lower eyelid is drawn down slightly, and the medication is instilled into the lower fornix, the nurse ensuring that the dropper or nozzle does not come into contact with the eye (Fig. 3.14). The patient is asked to close his eye and any excess medication is gently wiped away. If one tube of ointment is to be used for more than one patient, it is necessary to use glass rods to instil each patient's medication in order to prevent cross-contamination. Any signs of allergy to the medication, such as stinging of the skin, must be reported at once and recorded in the patient's notes.

Hot spoon bathing is commonly used as a treatment for styes and other inflammatory conditions of the eyelid. Since almost boiling water is used, the patient should be well supervised

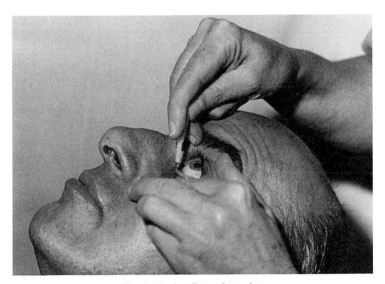

Fig. 3.14 *Instilling of eye drops.*

throughout the treatment in order to avoid scalding accidents. Requirements are:

> Jug or bowl containing almost boiling water
> Padded wooden spoon
> Protection for patient's clothing
> Sterile wool balls
> Disposal bag

The patient is seated at a table with his clothing protected. He is asked to dip the padded end of the spoon into the water and to allow surplus water to drain off. He is then instructed to lean slightly forward, close his eyes, and bring the spoon close to his eyelids, though avoiding direct contact. The heat from the padded spoon will cause vasodilation in the eyelids, increasing blood flow to them. Treatment should be continued for about 20 minutes, with as many changes of water as necessary. It may be prescribed four or more times a day. When treatment is completed, the patient's eyelids should be dried with cotton wool and the protective coverings removed. Small hot pads may be used as an alternative.

Cutting eyelashes is necessary prior to ophthalmic surgery since they cannot be adequately sterilized. It may also be carried out if the lashes are distorted by burns or if they contain lice. In addition to equipment for bathing the eye, the nurse will need a sharp pair of blunt-ended scissors and some white petroleum jelly. A good light source must be available. The patient should be seated or lying with his head well supported, as he must keep very still during this procedure. Petroleum jelly should be wiped on the scissor blades using a piece of gauze. The patient will then be asked to look down while the nurse, standing behind him, draws up the upper lid and cuts the upper eyelashes close to the lid margin. The eyelashes will adhere to the greased blades, which should be wiped and re-greased from time to time. The lower eyelashes are trimmed while the patient looks up. The fornices must be checked for fallen lashes before the patient is left.

Taking conjunctival cultures will be necessary prior to intraocular surgery to ensure that no infection is present, or if the causative organism of any eye or orbit infection needs to be identified. A sterile swab stick, transport medium and the appropriate request form will be needed. The patient is seated with his head well supported. After washing her hands, the nurse asks the patient to look up, gently draws down his lower lid and draws the swab along the exposed conjunctiva of the lower fornix from the medial side to the lateral. Great care must be taken not to contaminate the swab by touching the surrounding skin or lashes. The swab is then placed in the transport medium, labelled clearly with all necessary details, including which eye the swab is from, and sent to the laboratory.

Lacrimal sac washout may be necessary to establish patency of the tear ducts. The procedure is uncomfortable though not painful, and the patient should be warned of this and informed that local anaesthetic drops will be used to lessen the discomfort. In addition to equipment for bathing the eye, the nurse will need:

> Two Nettleship dilators (Fig. 3.15)
> 2 ml syringe
> Two lacrimal cannulae
> Gutt. Benoxinate 0.4% or Amethocaine 1%

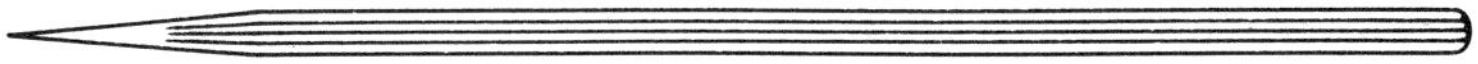

Fig. 3.15 *The Nettleship dilator.*

After bathing the patient's eye, the nurse should anaesthetize it with the local anaesthetic. She should then fill the syringe with sterile normal saline and attach the lacrimal cannula. She should stand behind the patient, draw his lower lid slightly down and laterally, and introduce the dilator to the punctum, gently rotating it between her thumb and finger as she does so. It should be passed vertically for about 2 mm and then turned horizontally to follow the path of the canaliculus. The nurse should remove the dilator and introduce the cannula along the same path (Fig. 3.16), passing it about 7 or 8 mm horizontally before gently depressing the plunger. If the passage is patent, the fluid will run down the back of the patient's throat causing him to cough. He should be advised to swallow the fluid and asked about its taste. If the duct is blocked, it will be difficult to depress the syringe plunger. Any fluid, pus or mucus flowing back through the upper punctum should be noted.

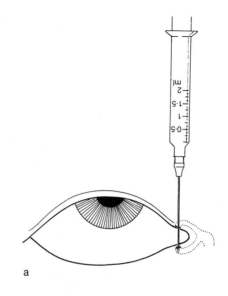

a

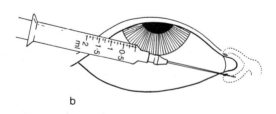

b

Fig. 3.16 *Syringing of the lacrimal passages. (a) Inserting the lacrimal cannula into the punctum. (b) Passing the lacrimal cannula along the canaliculus: when in position the passages are flushed with saline solution.*

Antibiotics may be instilled using this technique when infection is present in the canaliculus.

Subconjunctival injection of mydriatics may be necessary to dilate the pupil prior to or following surgery. It is also necessary to break down posterior synechiae, and steroids may be necessary to combat inflammation in patients with anterior uveitis. Concentrated antibiotics may be injected when intra-ocular infection is present. In addition to eye bathing equipment, the following will be required;

> Local anaesthetic drops
> 2 ml syringe and needles size 21G and 25G
> Prescription sheet and prescribed drug
> Bandage and adhesive tape

The patient should be assured that local anaesthetic will be used and that he will feel no pain, although he will experience a sensation of fullness within his eye as the drug is injected. The patient's eye should be bathed and anaesthetized using the local anaesthetic four times at five-minute intervals. The drug to be given is checked against the prescription sheet and drawn up into the syringe, the fine bore (25G) needle is attached and all air bubbles expelled. The patient is asked to look up and the nurse draws his lower lid down before inserting the needle horizontally under the bulbar conjunctiva, low in the fornix from the lateral side towards the medial. The medication should be injected slowly. Once the needle is removed, the patient is asked to close his eye, and this is padded and bandaged gently. Any prescribed analgesic should be given.

Rodding of the fornices is normally carried out to prevent or break down symblepharon (adhesions between lid and eyeball) which can follow a burn to the eye. In addition to equipment for bathing the eye, the following will be needed:

> Glass rod without chips or cracks
> Prescription sheet and prescribed medication
> Local anaesthetic drops

This treatment is uncomfortable, and it is essential that the eye is adequately anaesthetized and that the patient is given a full explanation of the need to carry out the procedure.

The nurse should bathe the eye as normal. She should then smear the end of the glass rod liberally with the prescribed ointment. The patient is asked to look up, the lower eyelid is drawn slightly down and the rod is directed vertically into the lower fornix and swept across it three or four times. The rod is re-greased and the process is repeated with the upper lid, the patient being asked to look down. Any excess ointment should be removed from the patient's lids.

The patient will be left with a film of ointment between his lids and eyeball, and should be instructed to move his eyes in all directions frequently between treatments.

FURTHER READING

Garland, P. (1975) *Ophthalmic Nursing*, 6th Edn. London: Faber and Faber.

4 The eyelids

Osondu Ibe was involved in a car accident while returning from holiday with his parents. No-one was seriously injured but Oson-du's eyelids were badly lacerated and needed surgical repair. He was an extremely difficult 14-year-old, who would not understand the need for admission to hospital and was obstreperous and unco-operative.

The following day, once he had recovered from the general anaesthetic, Osondu was a changed character, courteous to every-one and a great help in the ward. His eyelids were very painful, particularly when bathed and when his eye drops were instilled, but he grinned cheerfully, well able to cope now that his fear and shock had subsided.

STRUCTURE OF THE EYELIDS

The eyelids are mobile folds of tissue which protect the anterior surface of the eyeball. The upper eyelid merges with the skin of the eyebrow and the lower with the skin of the cheek. The thin skin is continuous at the lid margins with the conjunctiva which lines the eyelids (Fig. 4.1). A grey line, situated just behind the eyelashes, divides the anterior and posterior portions of the eyelids.

The tarsal plates give the eyelids their shape and firmness. They consist of dense fibrous and some elastic tissue and are continuous with the orbital septum. The meibomian glands within the tarsal plate secrete sebum which lubricates the eyelid margins, restrains tear overflow and prevents over-evaporation of tears from the surface of the cornea.

The eyelashes are inserted into the loose connective tissue and muscle of the anterior lip. The sweat glands of Moll open near the lashes, while the sebaceous glands of Zeis are attached directly to the eyelash follicles.

Two muscles are responsible for opening and closing the lids. The *orbicularis oculi* or sphincter muscle is striate muscle supplied by the facial nerve (VIIth cranial) and is responsible for closing

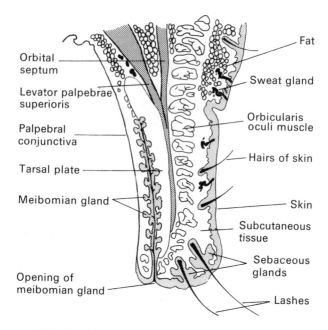

Fig. 4.1 *Longitudinal section through the upper eyelid.*

the eyelid. The palpebral portion affects the blink reflex, normal blink rate being every three to five seconds, while the orbital portion is used to close the eyes tightly. Horner's muscle is part of the orbicularis muscle which aids the drainage of tears by pulling on the lacrimal sac during blinking, thus creating a vacuum which draws tears into the sac. The muscle of Riolan is that part of the orbicularis oculi which occupies almost the whole thickness of the lid margin. The *levator palpebra superioris*, a voluntary muscle supplied by the oculomotor nerve (IIIrd cranial), acts to raise the upper lid.

The blood supply to the eyelids is derived mainly from the ophthalmic and lacrimal arteries. The veins are larger and more numerous than the arteries and empty into the veins of the forehead and temple, as well as into the ophthalmic vein.

The gap between the upper and lower eyelid is known as the palpebral fissure (Fig. 4.2) and ends at the inner and outer canthi. At the inner canthus is a small rounded structure called the caruncle. Beside the caruncle is a small elevated area, the papilla

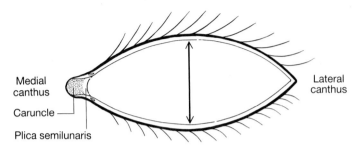

Fig. 4.2 *Palpebral fissure.*

lacrimalis, which is pierced by the punctum lacrimale, the entrance to the tear or lacrimal drainage system.

The eyebrows are thickened ridges of mobile skin covered with short hairs. They cover the superior orbital ridges. Many muscles of facial expression are attached to the eyebrows so that they may be raised, lowered or drawn towards the midline. They protect the eyes from perspiration and trap organic and inorganic matter.

FUNCTIONS OF THE EYELIDS

(1) To protect the eyeball by blinking and closure.
(2) To spread tears over the anterior surface of the cornea to keep it moist.
(3) To suppress visual stimuli, e.g. during sleep.
(4) To assist lacrimal drainage by blinking.
(5) To retard evaporation of tears from cornea by secretion from meibomian glands.
(6) To provide oxygen for the cornea from palpebral conjunctival artery.

DISEASES OF THE EYELIDS

CONGENITAL AND ACQUIRED

Ablepharon, or absence of eyelids, is a rare condition sometimes associated with absence of the eyeball. Early reconstruction surgery is essential to preserve the eyeball.

Coloboma is a notch, usually in the centre of the upper eyelid. Surgery to reconstruct the lid is necessary to prevent damage to the cornea from drying.

Epicanthus is a perpendicular fold of skin covering the medial canthus and is normally bilateral (Fig. 4.3). The condition may be familial and is characteristic of mongoloid races and sufferers of Down's syndrome. It is associated with a broad nasal bridge and gives the appearance of a convergent squint. If the condition persists and is unsightly, plastic surgery can be performed to remove the epicanthus.

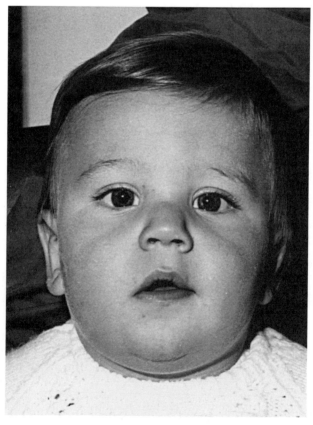

Fig. 4.3 *An epicanthic fold simulating squint.*

Distichiasis is a condition in which an extra row of eyelashes is present on the inner edge of the eyelid margin (Fig. 4.4); these continuously rub on the front of the eye. Some patients have been successfully treated by electrolysis but surgery to the eyelids is the only really satisfactory method of treatment.

Trichiasis (Fig. 4.4) is a common condition in which the eyelashes grow backwards and irritate the cornea and conjunctiva. Epilation (removal) of the lashes should be performed in the first instance, but for those patients whose lashes continue to recur in the abnormal position, electrolysis is recommended.

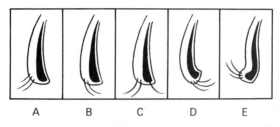

Fig. 4.4 *Section of the upper eyelid showing normal and abnormal positions of the tarsus and lashes. A, Normal eyelid; B, trichiasis; C, distichiasis; D, entropion; E, ectropion.*

Malposition of the eyelids may occur as either entropion or ectropion. *Entropion* is the rolling in of the eyelid margins (Fig. 4.4), most commonly the lower, with resultant discomfort as the eyelashes rub against the cornea. The condition may occur as a result of spasm or loss of tone in the orbicularis oculi muscle or following scarring of the conjunctiva lining the eyelids. A strip of adhesive tape applied from the lower eyelid to the cheek will keep the patient comfortable until surgery can be performed.

Ectropion is the turning outwards of the eyelids (Fig. 4.4), with the result that the tears are unable to drain. They collect at the lower fornix, stagnate and cause conjunctivitis. The eyelid appears to have a red rim of raw flesh and can be unsightly. Paralysis or loss of tone of the orbicularis oculi muscle are common causes of ectropion, especially in the elderly, or it may result from scarring of the eyelids or surrounding skin. Cautery to the conjunctiva just inside the lid margin may cure the condition if mild, but otherwise surgery is required.

Ptosis is drooping of the upper eyelid and may be unilateral or bilateral, congenital or acquired. Congenital ptosis may be hereditary and is usually apparent at birth. In severe cases where the ptosis covers the pupil, there may be reduced vision (amblyopia). The levator muscle is usually defective and surgical treatment aims at shortening it. Everbusch's operation approaches the muscle through the skin, while in Blaskovic's operation the approach is through the conjunctiva. Another procedure involves attaching the frontalis muscle to the tarsal plate so that it raises the eyelid. Where possible, surgery is delayed until the child is five years old, but where the eyelid is covering the pupil surgery may be necessary earlier lest the eye become amblyopic.

Acquired ptosis is often bilateral and may be seen in patients with myasthenia gravis, muscular dystrophy or nerve injury or lesions. Surgery is not indicated; rather, the precipitating cause of the ptosis is treated.

Lagophthalmos is an inadequate closure of the eyelid due to facial paralysis, proptosis or lid retraction. The resulting exposure of the cornea may lead to drying, corneal ulcers or even perforation. Treatment is with artificial tears or ointment, but tarsorrhaphy may be necessary.

INFLAMMATORY DISEASES

Blepharitis, inflammation of the eyelid margin, may be either squamous or ulcerative. Squamous blepharitis is commonly caused by seborrhoea and is often seen in children and adolescents. The eyelid margins become swollen and red, and rubbing them aggravates the condition. The seborrhoea must be treated and an antibiotic ointment may be rubbed with a fingertip into the eyelid margin. Ulcerative blepharitis is usually due to a staphylococcal infection, the cause of which must be treated. The lashes become crusted and may fall out or turn inwards (trichiasis) and irritate the cornea. The crusts must be swabbed from the eyelid margins using a weak solution of sodium bicarbonate before antibiotic ointment is applied.

Patients should be taught proper lid hygiene. Excessive use of eye make-up may also exacerbate this condition.

A *hordeolum or stye* is an abscess in the glands of Zeis, which results in a localized hard tender swelling (Fig. 4.5). It may on occasions be the result of lowered resistance to infection, for example in the diabetic patient. Any precipitating cause must be treated. Hot spoon bathing (p. 31) will help bring the stye to a head, when it will usually discharge spontaneously or resolve. An antibiotic ointment will be prescribed. Removal of the appropriate eyelash may be necessary if the stye persists, but it should never be incised.

A *chalazion or meibomian cyst* is a cystic swelling which results when a meibomian gland becomes blocked with sebaceous material. It may present as a rounded swelling in the upper or lower eyelid (Fig. 4.6) which may cause corneal irritation. Occasionally, the chalazion will fibrose leaving a permanent hard nodule.

A small cyst may resolve spontaneously. A larger cyst will require incision and evacuation, a short surgical procedure normally performed in the out-patient theatre. Hot spoon bathing

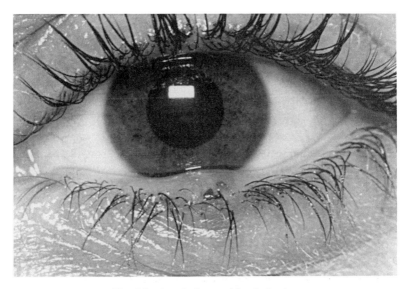

Fig. 4.5 *A style (external hordeolum).*

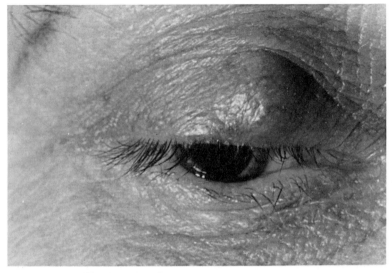

Fig. 4.6 *A meibomian cyst (internal hordeolum).*

and antibiotic ointment may be used where acute infection is present.

Cellulitis may result from many causes including trauma. allergies, injection. The underlying cause should always be treated. Systemic antibiotics may be necessary and incision and drainage should be carried out if a septic area does not rupture spontaneously.

TUMOURS OF THE EYELID

Benign tumours such as dermoid cysts, xanthelasmata, papillomata and molluscum contagiosum are usually removed surgically. Electrolysis, diathermy or electric cautery are the method of choice, although larger tumours may require dissection.

Malignant tumours

Rodent ulcer (basal cell carcinoma) is the commonest of the malignant tumours of the eyelid. It occurs more commonly on the lower eyelid and near to the lid margin. The ulcer has a raised edge with an ulcerated centre which tends to bleed; it may be pigmented. Neglected ulcers can invade the orbit and cranial cavity, but it is of low malignancy and does not metastasize.

Squamous cell carcinoma, sarcoma and *malignant melanoma* are all rare tumours of the eyelid.

Diagnosis of all malignant tumours must be confirmed by biopsy. If surgical removal is the treatment of choice, a rim of about 3 mm of healthy skin is removed with the tumour. Skin or mucous membrane grafts may be necessary. Many tumours are satisfactorily treated with radiotherapy, a lead contact lens being use to protect the eye while treatment is administered.

INJURIES TO THE EYELID

Blunt injuries to the eyelids cause bruising and swelling where fluid leaks into the loose subdermal tissues. Immediately applied cold compresses may lessen the bleeding.

Penetrating wounds of the eyelid require careful surgical repair, particularly if the wound is in the area of the canaliculi. Early repair should be performed in tears through the lid margin in order to prevent trichiasis and epiphora.

NURSING CONSIDERATIONS

- Following some forms of corrective surgery to the eyelids, notably for ptosis, the patient may need re-education regarding correct positioning of the head. Most patients will have tilted their heads to overcome the problem.
- Where sutures are inserted through the lower eyelid to keep the eyelids closed, the ends are left long and drawn upwards where they are taped to the forehead.
- Following suture removal, the palpebral fissure should be observed while the patient is asleep to ensure that the cornea is not exposed, since this will lead to a drying out of the corneal epithelium with subsequent infection and ulceration and the complications thereof.
- If the eyelids are not properly closed in sleep, antibiotic ointment is instilled to lubricate and protect the cornea and prevent

drying. The patient may need to be taught to do this himself, and the reason should be fully explained to and understood by the patient.

- Pads should not be applied when the lids do not meet properly, as they may cause corneal abrasion.
- It is normal procedure to insert many fine sutures in the eyelids in order to prevent skin puckering and scarring. The sutures must be kept clean and free of crusting so that tissue loss when they are removed is minimized.
- When tarsorrhaphy (suturing together of the lids) is performed, rubber tubing is often used to act as a splint to the lid margins and to prevent puckering (Fig. 4.7). This must be fully explained to the patient, and special care will be needed when removing the sutures.
- It must not be forgotten that even apparently minor surgery which results in temporary loss of vision will affect the patient's ability to care for himself as he would normally do, and nursing intervention may be necessary in the performance of many daily activities.

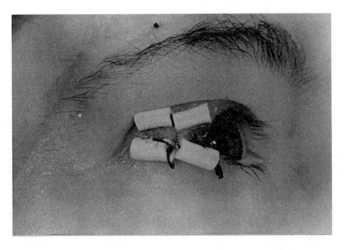

Fig. 4.7 *Tarsorrhaphy with rubber tubes. The rubber tubes hold the eyelid edges together until they heal. Only one suture may be necessary with each set of tubes.*

FURTHER READING

Perkins, E.S., Hansell, P. & Marsh, R.J. (1986) *An Atlas of Diseases of the Eye*, 3rd Edn. Edinburgh: Churchill Livingstone.

Trevor-Roper, P.D. (1980) *Lecture Notes on Ophthalmology*, 6th Edn. Oxford: Blackwell Scientific.

Vaughan, D. & Asbury, T. (1974) *General Ophthalmology*, 7th Edn. Los Altos, California: Lange Medical Publications.

5 The orbit

Hector Brown staggered into Casualty one February morning, clearly the worse from drink and looking somewhat dishevelled. He had fallen two days previously, hitting his head, and now was almost unable to see. Examination revealed bilateral lacerations to the eyebrows which had become infected, and were discharging pus and causing severe orbital cellulitis. He was extremely ill and was admitted to the ward for urgent treatment.

STRUCTURE OF THE ORBITS

The orbits are four-sided pyramids situated on either side of the nose with their apices directed backwards and inwards. Each orbit is composed of seven bones, three of which (the frontal, ethmoid and sphenoid bones) are common to both, and four of which (zygoma, maxillary, palatine and lacrimal) are individual (Fig. 5.1). The anterior margin of the orbital cavity is thickened to provide protection for the eye, but the walls of the orbit are very thin, particularly the medial wall and the floor.

BONES

The roof or vault of the orbit is triangular in shape and is formed by the orbital plate of the frontal bone and the lesser wing of the sphenoid. The bone is translucent and thin and easily fractured by direct violence. In the elderly, portions of the roof may be absorbed so that the peri-orbital space is in direct contact with the dura mater.

The orbit's lateral wall is formed of the zygomatic (malar) bone and the greater wing of the sphenoid. It is triangular in shape with its base anteriorly. The superior and inferior orbital fissures separate the sphenoidal portion from the roof and floor. It is the thickest of the walls and the most exposed to injury.

The superior maxillary bone, lacrimal, ethmoid and sphenoid bones form the oblong medial walls which are parallel to one

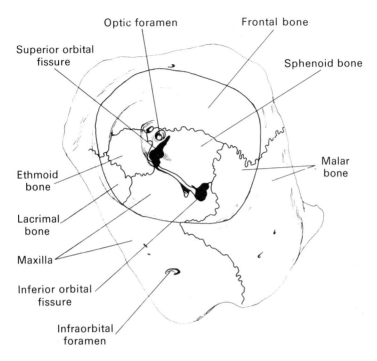

Fig. 5.1 *Bones forming the left orbit.*

another. These are the thinnest of the walls (0.2–0.4 mm) and are translucent. Infection from the ethmoidal air cells of the nasal antrum can easily cross into the orbits via the medial walls, and ethmoiditis is the commonest cause of orbital cellulitis. The orbital floor is formed mainly by the orbital plate of the superior maxilla with the palatine and zygomatic bones. The antrum of Highmore (maxillary sinus) lies directly below the floor, and tumours of the antrum can easily cross the 0.5–1.0 mm of bone to invade the orbit, causing proptosis.

SINUSES

A number of other accessory sinuses surround the orbit: they all communicate with the nose and act to lighten the skull and give resonance to the voice. The frontal sinuses lie above the orbits and connect with the nose via the infundibulum, a narrow passage passing between the anterior ethmoidal air cells and entering the nose close to the openings of these cells and of the maxillary antrum. Infection in one sinus can and does spread readily to the others.

FORAMINA AND FISSURES

From the apex of each orbit a funnel-shaped optic foramen or optic canal leads to the middle cranial fossa. It is formed by the two roots of the lesser wing of the sphenoid and provides protection for the structures running through it, the optic nerve with its covering meninges (dura, arachnoid and pia mater), and the ophthalmic artery and vein which are embedded in the dural sheath of the optic nerve.

The superior orbital fissure lies between the roof and lateral wall of the orbit. The IIIrd, IVth, Vth and VIth cranial nerves (oculomotor, trochlear, trigeminal and abducens) enter through this fissure, and the superior and inferior ophthalmic veins leave through it to empty into the cavernous sinus of the cranium.

The inferior orbital, or spheno-maxillary, fissure lies between the lateral wall and the floor of the orbit. The maxillary division of the Vth cranial nerve, the zygomatic nerves and the ophthalmic vein pass through it.

The anterior and posterior ethmoidal foramina, lying between the roof and medial wall of the orbit, supply the sinuses with the ethmoidal artery and nerve. The infra-orbital artery and nerve (Vth cranial) are carried in the infra-orbital canal.

CONTENTS OF THE ORBIT

(1) The eyeball.
(2) Muscles: six extra-ocular plus the levator muscle of the eyelid.
(3) The lacrimal gland.
(4) The orbital fascia: the periosteum is in close contact with all the bones of the orbit.
(5) The orbital fat.
(6) The orbital blood vessels and nerves: ophthalmic veins have

no valves and drainage is influenced by gravity and head position. The orbital venous system links the cranial and facial systems.

FUNCTION OF THE ORBIT

The bones of the orbit provide protection from injury for their contents, particularly the eyeball. The bones are thickest at the orbital margin where the orbit joins the face and where direct traumatic injury is most likely to occur.

DISEASES OF THE ORBIT

Because the bony orbit is rigid it allows only anterior displacement of the globe if there is an increase in the orbital contents. Unilateral proptosis or bilateral exophthalmos is thus a principal sign of orbital disease.

INFLAMMATORY DISEASES

Orbital cellulitis is most commonly caused by direct bacterial infection from the ethmoid sinus, by a penetrating orbital injury or via the orbital veins from a focus of pus in the eyelids.

Anterior orbital cellulitis will lead to severe oedema of the lids and sometimes pointing of the inflammation through the skin of the lid. The conjunctiva may be injected and chemosed but the eyeball is unaffected and able to move freely.

Posterior orbital cellulitis is a serious condition in which proptosis of the eyeball results from a build-up of fluid in the orbit. Conjunctival chemosis is generally present and the eyelids become oedematous. The patient will experience severe pain, particularly when moving his eyes, as pressure affects the extra-ocular muscles. He will feel very unwell and will be pyrexial or even hyperpyrexial. If the condition is untreated, meningitis, cerebral abscess, optic neuritis or cavernous sinus thrombosis may ensue.

Cavernous sinus thrombosis is the most serious complication of orbital cellulitis, and is an acute thrombophlebitis of the cavernous sinus. Patients with this complication are extremely ill (about 50% die) because the focus of infection is isolated by the blood/brain barrier and is inaccessible for surgical drainage. The patient will present with a severe headache or may be comatose. The ophthalmic muscles and nerves are usually involved, resulting in papilloedema and visual failure. Proptosis is common.

The patient with orbital cellulitis will be admitted to hospital and all possible precautions taken to prevent cross-infection. A nursing assessment will highlight the many areas in which such an acutely ill patient will need help with his daily activities, but attention to hydration and personal cleansing will be high priorities. Intravenous fluids may be necessary if dehydration is to be avoided and the nurse should ensure that the patient receives adequate analgesia. Conjunctival swabs should be taken prior to the commencement of intensive broad-spectrum antibiotic therapy, which may be used both topically and systemically. Hot spoon bathing (see p. 31) may help to ease the discomfort. The patient's temperature, pulse and respiratory rate will be closely monitored. Anticoagulants may be prescribed if cavernous venous thrombosis is suspected. Once the cause of the cellulitis has been diagnosed, specific treatment may be indicated; for example, incision and drainage of an infected nasal sinus or abscess.

TRAUMATIC INJURY

Orbital fractures

Orbital fractures and dislocations are commonly associated with other facial fractures, head injuries and severe lacerations. They are usually recognizable on X-ray and often cause ecchymosis and conjunctival haemorrhage. Orbital fractures generally heal without active intervention.

A *blowout fracture* results when the blow to the eyeball causes such a rise in intra-orbital pressure that the orbital contents are forced through the orbital floor and herniate into the ethmoidal sinus or air cells. The eyeball sinks inwards (enophthalmos), although bruising may mask this sign initially, and the patient is unable to rotate his eye upwards if the extra-ocular muscles are trapped in the hernia. These fractures require surgical repair only if there is diplopia and permanent restriction of eye movement, suggesting incarceration of orbital tissue in the fracture.

Retrobulbar haemorrhage

This most commonly results from direct injuries tearing the periosteal blood vessels. It may also occur in haemorrhagic or arterial diseases and in any venous congestion which involves all the veins of the head and neck as in strangulation.

Proptosis is apparent in proportion to the severity of the haemorrhage and the blood may track to appear subconjunctivally. Pain is usually present and ocular movement may be limited.

The haemorrhage will normally resolve spontaneously within a few weeks, although incision and drainage of the orbit are occasionally indicated.

METABOLIC DISORDERS

Thyroid disease will be covered in Chapter 18.

Horner's syndrome occurs when damage to the cervical sympathetic nerve causes the triad of miosis (constriction of the pupil), partial ptosis and enophthalmos. The syndrome may result from a number of lesions such as pressure from carcinoma of branches occurring in the region of the cervical ganglion. It may occur following operations on the thyroid gland or as a result of aortic aneurysm. Treatment may involve surgery to deal with the ptosis (see Chapter 4).

ORBITAL TUMOURS

Primary tumours may arise in a number of orbital contents: bone (osteosarcoma); muscle (rhabdomyosarcoma); optic nerve (glioma, meningioma); lacrimal gland (adenoma, adenocarcinoma); connective tissue (fibroma, neurofibromatosis); or blood vessels (haemangioma).

Secondary deposits from adjacent structures and metastatic deposits are less commonly found.

Diplopia is a common early sign of displacement of the eyeball (proptosis) which may be marked. Congestion and oedema of the eyelids and conjunctiva are usual. Bruit in the head, such as the sound of running water, can be the most annoying symptom of a tumour. Folds may appear in the choroid and papilloedema may be present if venous drainage is compromised.

Diagnosis is now generally made using ultrasound or computerized tomography.

Surgical removal or orbital tumours may be achieved without significant damage to the eye, but may have to involve exenteration of the orbital contents, enucleation of the eye and correction of any bony defects. Chemotherapy and/or radiotherapy may be used instead of, or in addition to, any surgical procedures.

NURSING CONSIDERATIONS

- The importance of individual assessment cannot be over-stressed, particularly when dealing with the acutely ill patient. Hector Brown (see profile) had masked his symptoms with alcohol, was unable to appreciate the fact that he was extremely ill, and was most reluctant to remain in his single room. Another patient with the same degree of cellulitis might be prostrate and require intensive support.
- The patient should be offered analgesics at regular intervals, and nursing assessment will evaluate its effect. Most patients will require help with such activities as personal cleansing and feeding. In the early stages of the illness, nursing intervention should aim at maintaining the patient's hydration as most will feel too ill to eat.
- In severe cases of orbital cellulitis where there is abscess formation and increasing proptosis, it may be necessary to record the patient's visual acuity hourly. The need for surgical intervention would be indicated by a deterioration in the patient's general condition accompanied by worsening visual acuity. Following incision and drainage, visual acuity usually improves rapidly.
- Maximum physical and mental comfort should be aimed for when nursing the acutely ill ophthalmic patient. Many patients find that bright light increases their pain and that the constant visual stimuli provided in an open ward are difficult to ignore.

Most will recover more quickly if nursed in a single ward with the curtains drawn, so that the eyes may be rested as much as possible. Boredom can be alleviated by listening to the radio or a talking book if this is available.

- Where fractures of the orbit are associated with other injuries, the danger of the patient's becoming shocked must not be forgotten (see Chapter 15).
- Rapid loss of vision following orbital fracture may indicate retrobulbar haemorrhage and should always be pointed out. Such haemorrhage would require drainage.
- Where severe proptosis or exophthalmos is present, it is important to keep the cornea lubricated and protected. Tarsorrhaphy may be necessary if artificial tears and ointment are inadequate, as it is essential to prevent damage to the cornea. An alternative is to apply a clear Perspex bubble which adheres to the skin of the orbital area enclosing the front of the eye. Pads must *not* be applied.

FURTHER READING

Miller, S.J.H. (1984) *Parsons' Diseases of the Eye*, 17th Edn. Edinburgh: Churchill Livingstone.

Perkins, E.S., Hansell, P. & Marsh, R.J. (1986) *An Atlas of Diseases of the Eye*, 3rd Edn. Edinburgh: Churchill Livingstone.

Sachsenweger, R. (1980) *Illustrated Handbook of Ophthalmology*. Bristol: John Wright.

6 The conjunctiva

Fiona had been unable to open her eyes. They had been sticky with pus when she woke on the two previous days but this morning it had taken several minutes of bathing with warm water before her lids would separate. By the time she was seen in the eye department, her facial skin was sore from the pus that constantly flowed from her eyes. Irrigation of her eyes for 20 minutes was necessary before she could be examined properly.

Conjunctivitis was diagnosed and conjunctival swabs were taken to confirm this. Chloramphenicol eye drops 0.5% were instilled into both her eyes every half hour for the next 3 hours, while she remained in the department. She was allowed to leave only when the nurses were sure she could instil the drops correctly.

Fiona's eyes soon felt less uncomfortable and her strict adherence to the intensive treatment regime ensured that the condition resolved completely, fortunately without long-term complications.

STRUCTURE OF THE CONJUNCTIVA

The conjunctiva is a thin, transparent mucous membrane which lines the posterior surface of the eyelids and is reflected forward onto the globe of the eye, becoming continuous anteriorly with the corneal epithelium. The conjunctiva thus forms a potential sac, open at the palpebral fissure (Fig. 6.1). Goblet cells within the epithelial layer of the conjunctiva secrete mucin which forms part of the tear film. The accessory lacrimal glands of Krause and Wolfring are located deep in the conjunctiva's stromal layer.

The palpebral portion of the conjunctiva is that which lines the eyelids and is continuous with the skin of the eyelids at the lid margins. The membrane is thin and very vascular and the meibomian glands are visible through it as yellowish streaks. The palpebral conjunctiva is connected via the puncta and lacrimal passages to the inferior meatus of the nose, and diseases in one may spread to the other.

The fornices are continuous circular cul-de-sacs broken only by the caruncles and plicae semilunaris. The caruncle is a small

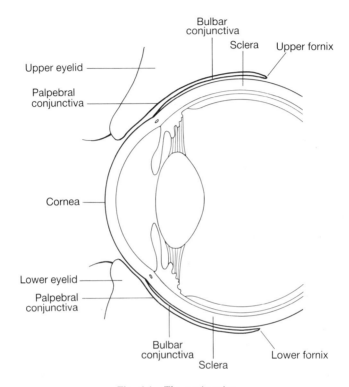

Bulbar conjunctiva
Sclera
Upper fornix
Upper eyelid
Palpebral conjunctiva
Cornea
Lower eyelid
Palpebral conjunctiva
Bulbar conjunctiva
Sclera
Lower fornix

Fig. 6.1 *The conjunctiva.*

fleshy-looking ovoid body and is attached to the narrow crescentic fold of conjunctiva known as the plica semilunaris (see Fig. 4.2). The plica represents the third eyelid or nictitating membrane of the lower animals (readily visible in cats and dogs).

The bulbar portion of the conjunctiva covers the eyeball and is so thin and transparent that the white sclera is visible through it. The membrane lies loosely on the underlying tissues and is easily separated from them.

The conjunctiva has a rich blood supply derived from the palpebral arteries of the lids and the anterior ciliary arteries. The more numerous veins drain into the anterior ciliary veins. Nerve supply to the conjunctiva is from the same source as that of the eyelids.

FUNCTIONS OF THE CONJUNCTIVA

(1) To moisturize and lubricate the cornea.
(2) To protect the underlying sclera.
(3) To prevent the entry of foreign bodies, organisms and other noxious substances into the orbit.
(4) To allow extreme movement of the eyeball.
(5) To assist in the re-epithelialization of the cornea if this should be scraped or burned.

DISEASES OF THE CONJUNCTIVA

Most patients with conjunctival disease will complain of ocular discomfort or burning, with or without exudation. Itching is common in allergic conditions but severe pain suggests secondary corneal involvement. Inflammatory exudate may cause excoriation of the skin, particularly at the outer canthus, or cause the eyelids to stick together during sleep. A noteworthy feature is the absence of pain as a presenting feature.

CONJUNCTIVITIS

This is an inflammation of the conjunctiva which is characterized by cellular infiltration and exudation. The eye looks red or pink. Conjunctivitis may be caused by bacteria, viruses, fungi, parasites, toxins, chemicals, foreign bodies or allergens and may be acute, sub-acute or chronic. Infectious conjunctivitis is often bilateral due to cross-infection, and other members of the family or friends may be involved. Copious exudate is usually indicative of bacterial infections, while stringy, sparse exudate suggests an allergy or viral infection. Diagnosis will be made from the history and clinical examination, but conjunctival scrapings and swabs should be taken in order to identify the cause.

Acute conjunctivitis

The patient will usually present with a red, discharging eye which burns and feels 'gritty'. The discharge may be watery, mucopurulent or purulent depending on the causative organism. The condition will spread readily to the other eye and care must be taken to prevent this. Antibiotic eyedrops are normally prescribed once swabs and sometimes scrapings have been taken. These should be instilled at least four times daily.

Saline irrigation may be necessary if the discharge contains pus. Mucopurulent discharge is common in acute fevers such as measles and scarlet fever, while purulent discharge is due to bacterial infection. In the latter case there is a real risk of corneal involvement, with devitalization and ulceration of the corneal epithelium. Systemic antibiotics may be required in addition to the prescribed antibiotic eye drops and ointment. The nurse must be very careful to maintain high standards of hygiene when dealing with these patients, and to ensure that they understand the importance of the measures taken to avoid cross-infection.

Ophthalmia neonatorum is a form of acute conjunctivitis often transmitted during birth (Fig. 6.2). If the discharge commences

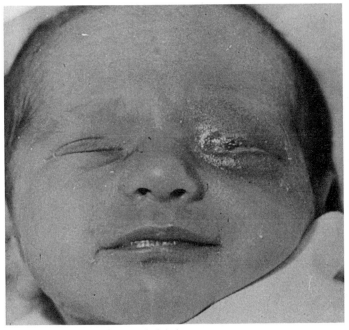

Fig. 6.2 *Ophthalmia neonatorum.*

within 21 days of birth, the medical staff are required to notify the health authority. Usually both eyes are involved; the lids may be swollen, the conjunctiva is red and often chemosed and there is mucopurulent or purulent discharge. Common causative organisms are gonococcus, Chlamydia (TRIC) and pneumococcus. In severe cases the cornea becomes involved and perforation may result. Treatment will be an intensive regime of antibiotic eye drops, with systemic antibiotics if necessary, and atropine drops if the cornea is involved. Again, the nurse must take great care not to be the agent of cross-infection.

Photophthalmia is a violent conjunctival reaction secondary to oedema of the corneal epithelium: it is caused by exposure to ultra-violet light. Photophthalmia most commonly occurs when unprotected eyes are exposed to the light of arc welding, electric flashes or sunlit snowfields (snow blindness). It may also occur following the use of 'arc lamps' without the wearing of protective goggles. There is a delay of several hours between exposure and the onset of symptoms, which include intense burning pain, copious tear production and photophobia. It is often impossible for the sufferer to open his eyes (see also Chapter 15).

Chronic conjunctivitis

This results from exposure to some form of irritant; a concretion, trichiasis, dust, smoke, infection from the lacrimal sac or nasal catarrh are common causes. Some drugs, notably atropine, pilocarpine, eserine, and animal dander, particularly from horses and cats, act as allergic stimuli in some people.

Chronic conjunctivitis may follow an acute episode or be characterized by recurrent attacks. Treatment is with local antibiotic and steroid therapy. Dark glasses may help some patients by reducing glare. Where possible, the cause should be eliminated.

Viral conjunctivitis

Viral disease is a cause of conjunctivitis and is often due to adenovirus or *Herpes simplex*.

The adenovirus usually affects both eyes and the onset is acute with infection of the conjunctiva. This is a contagious condition, and outbreaks occur in places such as schools, offices or residential establishments.

There is no effective antiviral treatment, but antibiotic drops may usually be used to prevent secondary bacterial infection.

Herpes simplex is also an acute infection with follicular conjunctivitis. *Herpes simplex* conjunctivitis is usually unilateral. Antiviral treatment may be used. These patients usually complain of their eyes watering and nipping, but they are not sticky.

Conjunctival swabs and scrapings are normally taken prior to the commencement of treatment.

Trachoma (inclusion conjunctivitis) is the most important cause of preventable blindness throughout the world. It occurs mainly in the developing countries of the Third World in which conditions and standards of hygiene are poor. The causative organism, *Chlamydia trachomatis*, may be spread by flies or in shared washing water or cosmetics. It is frequently accompanied by bacterial infection. Complex chains of infection and re-infection occur because of poor sanitation and large population of 'eye-seeking' flies. Trachoma was a serious public health hazard in this country 150 years ago, but has disappeared following legislation regarding water supplies and sewage disposal, better housing conditions, and many years of treatment with antibiotics.

Reiter's syndrome

This will be dealt with in Chapter 18.

DEGENERATIVE CHANGES

Pinguecula

This is the name given to small, yellow, triangular nodules which appear on either side of the cornea. They occur in middle age, especially in people who lead an outdoor life, and are probably caused by constant exposure to sunlight, wind or dust. They are symptomless and require no treatment.

Pterygium

A pterygium is a triangular fold of bulbar conjunctiva that advances over the cornea, most commonly from the nasal side (Fig. 6.3). The conjunctiva becomes thickened and very vascular

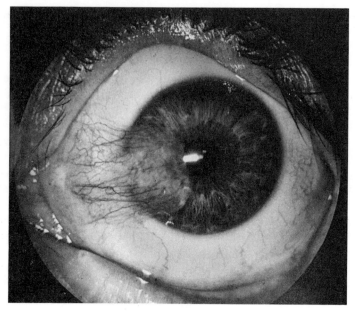

Fig. 6.3 *Pterygium.*

in response to chronic recurrent dryness at the corneo-scleral border. This occurs mainly in individuals who spend much of their time out of doors, especially in dry sunny countries, and it may cause discomfort. Corneal excision will be necessary if the pterygium grows over the cornea, as vision will be impaired if it reaches the pupil area.

TUMOURS OF THE CONJUNCTIVA

Benign tumours

Dermoid cysts usually occur at the corneo-scleral junction and may involve both of these structures. They consist of fibro-adipose tissue with epidermis, hair and sebaceous follicles, and are firmly fixed to the cornea. Surgical removal is recommended.

Pigmented naevus is situated near the limbus and is freely movable with the conjunctiva. They may be any shade of brown.

Removal may be necessary if the naevus appears to be developing malignant changes.

Granulomata and *papillomata* may occur in the conjunctiva. They should be removed with scissors and cauterized.

Malignant tumours

Malignant tumours may occur as papilloma (a 'raspberry' appearance), epithelioma ('cauliflower' appearance and easily ulcerates), sarcoma (from pigmented naevi) or a rodent ulcer (spread directly from the eyelids). The tumours spread by local invasion and secondary deposits are frequent. (Note that rodent ulcers do not metastasize.)

In the early stages, local removal of the tumour, shaving of the sclera and treatment of the tumour base with radiotherapy will be undertaken.

Enucleation of the eye may be necessary for more advanced tumours and for those in their later stages, and exenteration of the orbit should be considered in addition (i.e. removal of eyelids, eyeball and all other orbital contents).

CONJUNCTIVAL INJURIES

Subconjunctival haemorrhage

This occurs when a conjunctival blood vessel is ruptured. A bright red, sharply delineated area appears, surrounded by normal-looking conjunctiva. Trauma, severe bouts of coughing or sneezing, hypertension and blood disorders may all cause haemorrhage, but often no cause is identified. The haemorrhage is symptomless, though its appearance may be alarming, and gradually fades over about two weeks. Haemorrhage involving the entire conjunctiva may follow a fracture of one of the orbital bones or rupture of the posterior sclera.

Wounds

Wounds heal rapidly in the absence of infection. Foreign bodies should be removed and dirty or jagged conjunctival edges trimmed and sutured as necessary. Antibiotic drops or ointment may be prescribed.

Burns

Burns may result from chemicals, both acids and alkalis, or from hot material, e.g. molten plastic, being thrown or splashed into the eye. They can cause great ocular damage by symblepharon formation and corneal ulceration or necrosis. They are extremely painful and the patient will naturally be fearful of permanent loss of vision. Once the pH of the patient's tears has been checked, anaesthetic drops should be instilled and the eye irrigated with copious amounts of saline for at least 15 minutes in an attempt to dilute the causative substance. Wherever possible, the specific antidote should be used. This is normally a buffered phosphate solution for acid burns, or sodium versenate for lime or alkaline burns. The local poisons centre will be able to give more specific information.

When irrigation is complete, fluorescein staining of the cornea should be carried out and the patient admitted to hospital if there is corneal involvement. Antibiotic and steroid ointments may be prescribed. Rodding of the fornices is sometimes undertaken if symblepharon begins to form, and may need to be continued daily until the burns have healed.

Where burn damage is severe, the conjunctival sac may need to be re-formed with a mucous membrane graft.

NURSING CONSIDERATIONS

- The prime aim of nursing those patients with disorders of the conjunctiva is to enhance those functions of the membrane (see above) that have been impaired by disease.
- A sound understanding of the means by which infection is transmitted from one source to another is vital if cross-infection is to be avoided.
- The nurse must fulfil the important role of patient educator when caring for those patients with conjunctivitis. Hospital admission may be avoided because of the risk of infection being passed to other patients. It is vital that the patients understand,

before leaving the clinic, the need for high standards of personal cleanliness. They should not share face flannels or towels with others, as this will increase the risk of cross-infection. Disposable tissues should be used rather than handkerchiefs and pillowslips should be washed regularly if there is any sign of discharge onto them. They should be taught to instil their own medication and understand the importance of careful hand-washing both before (to avoid introducing further infection) and after (to ensure that any bacteria are removed from the hands) this is done.

- Those patients with conjunctival burns are usually extremely worried about the amount of permanent damage they might suffer, and the nurse must take care to express her sympathy and understanding of their fears while dealing efficiently with the burned tissue. It is unreasonable to take a lengthy nursing history from a frightened patient in pain. The time and place of the accident, how it happened and what the causative substance was are all the information needed before irrigation is commenced. The nurse should explain all procedures fully, repeating the explanations if necessary since the frightened patient will be unlikely to assimilate much of what is said. Irrigating the eye following a burn injury may be extremely uncomfortable for the patient.

- No attempt should be made to record the visual acuity of the patient with conjunctival burns until after irrigation is complete.

- The upper eyelid will need double everting to ensure that the fornix is completely clear of chemical and particulate matter.

- A careful history and accurate record of care is particularly important when a patient has been injured at work, since claims for industrial injury may not be immediately pursued, and precise details may have been forgotten if they were not documented at the time of injury. The occupational health department at the patient's place of work may have been involved in his care prior to his arrival at hospital and should be informed, where appropriate, of the outcome. In some instances, the patient may wish to contact and involve his trade union representative following an industrial accident. Wherever possible, the use of abbreviations and jargon which may be misinterpreted must be avoided, both in verbal and written accounts of the patient's care.

FURTHER READING

Bedford, M.A. (1979) *A Colour Atlas of Ocular Tumours*. London: Wolfe Medical
    Publications.
Martin-Doyle, J.L.C. (1975) *A Synopsis of Ophthalmology*. Bristol: John Wright.
Perkins, E.S., Hansell, P. & Marsh, R.J. (1986) *An Atlas of Diseases of the Eye*,
    3rd Edn. Edinburgh: Churchill Livingstone.
Trevor-Roper, P.D. (1974) *The Eye and its Disorders*, 3rd Edn. Oxford: Blackwell
    Scientific.

7 The extra-ocular muscles

Ben was inconsolable when he realized that his parents had crept out and left him in the hospital ward—he screamed, stamped, kicked and finally curled up on his bed with his teddy and sobbed himself to sleep. When his parents visited that afternoon he refused to speak to them. He was two and the only child of doting parents who hadn't felt able to explain about his squint and the need for an operation to correct it because they felt somehow guilty about it all. Staff Nurse sat down with Ben and his parents and explained about visiting theatre and how Ben and Teddy would need drops put into their eyes. Ben showed no sign of listening and his parents clearly thought it far too complicated for him to understand. Next morning Ben rushed across to Staff Nurse as soon as she came on duty and showed her Teddy who had a wet left eye; he explained that he was going to theatre when his mummy and daddy arrived and when he woke up, he would have eye drops too. He was very excited about it all.

STRUCTURE AND FUNCTIONS

Each eye is moved by the six extra-ocular muscles which attach it to the bony orbit. They enable us to use both eyes together to provide a good retinal image for transmission to the brain. There are four rectus and two oblique muscles (see Fig. 2.2).

The *medial rectus* originates at the apex of the orbit at the annulus of Zinn, and runs parallel to the medial orbital wall to insert into the sclera, 5 mm from the limbus (the corneo-scleral junction). It turns the eye towards the nose (adduction); it is the muscle of convergence.

The *lateral rectus* originates at the annulus of Zinn, and runs close to the lateral wall of the orbit before inserting into the sclera, 7 mm from the limbus. It turns the eyes outwards (abduction); the muscle of divergence.

The *superior rectus* muscle runs from the annulus of Zinn, close to the orbital roof and immediately below the levator muscle, to insert into the sclera 8 mm from the limbus. It acts to turn the eye upwards (elevation) and to rotate it towards the nose (intorsion).

The *inferior rectus* passes from the annulus of Zinn close to the floor of the orbit, to insert 6 mm from the limbus. It turns the eyeball downwards (depression) and rotates it away from the nose (extorsion).

The *superior oblique* is the longest of the extra-ocular muscles. It originates at the apex of the orbit and runs in the angle formed by the junction of the roof and medial wall of the orbit. Just short of the margin of the orbit the muscle passes through the cartilaginous *trochlear pulley* and then runs below the superior rectus in a posterior, lateral direction (Fig. 2.2). It inserts into the lateral surface of the sclera, posterior to the equator or midline of the eye. It acts to depress the gaze and intort the eye.

Table 7.1 *Functions of the extra-ocular muscles*

Muscle	Primary action	Secondary action
Medial rectus	Adduction	—
Lateral rectus	Abduction	—
Superior rectus	Elevation	Intorsion
Inferior rectus	Depression	Extorsion
Superior oblique	Depression	Intorsion
Inferior oblique	Elevation	Extorsion

The *inferior oblique*, the shortest of the muscles, arises from the orbital floor close to the anterior border. It passes under the inferior rectus to insert into the lateral side of the sclera posterior to the equator. It acts to elevate and extort the eye.

The extra-ocular muscles are supplied by the IIIrd (medial, superior and inferior recti, inferior oblique), IVth (superior oblique) and VIth (lateral rectus) cranial nerves. Blood supply is by branches of the ophthalmic artery.

The muscles are encased in fascia, known as Tenon's capsule, which extends over the sclera. In normal vision, both eyes look in the same direction with the lines of vision parallel. Different muscles will be used in each eye to achieve simultaneous versional movement—these are termed *yoke muscles* (see Fig. 7.1). An

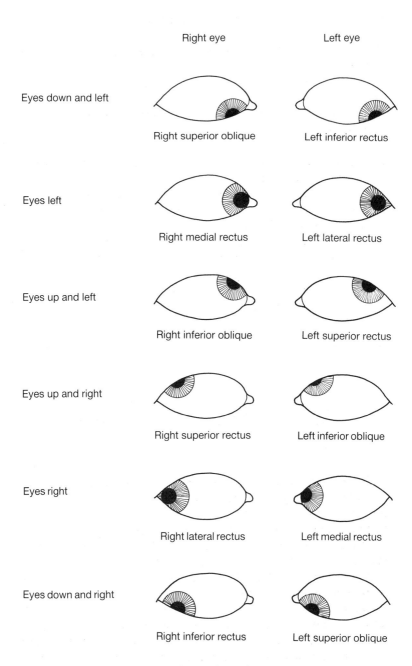

Fig. 7.1 *Yoke muscle combinations.*

equal innervational impulse flows from the cerebral oculogyric centres to each muscle involved (Hering's law) and a paretic muscle can be readily diagnosed by deviation of one eye when turned in the direction of the paralysed muscle. If the muscles are unbalanced or unsynchronized, binocular vision will be impaired because the macular area of highest visual acuity is small.

STRABISMUS

Strabismus (or squint) occurs when the extra-ocular muscles or the nerves supplying them are affected by disease or trauma. The visual axis of one eye or other deviates and a loss of parallel vision results. The deviation is usually in the horizontal plane and may be convergent or divergent. Squint may be accompanied by diplopia as the brain is unable to interpret the two sets of images presented to it.

MANIFEST SQUINT (heterotropia)

The manifest squint is one that is obvious. It may be intermittent or may exist only for certain distances of fusion (e.g. squint is manifest for distant fixation but not for near fixation).

The majority of squints are in the horizontal, although many are both horizontal and vertical.

It may be caused by uncorrected refractive errors, defective development of the visual pathways, ocular disease or febrile illness.

Concomitant squint is commonly seen in children. Each eye retains a normal range of movement and the same angle of deviation is present in all parts of the binocular field. The ability to use the two eyes together is not present at birth, but develops in the first year of life and is complete by the age of eight. The onset of squint will lead to diplopia because the eyes are no longer aligned. The child will learn to suppress the image seen by the deviant eye, and visual acuity in that eye will deteriorate causing amblyopia or a 'lazy' eye. The longer the squinting is allowed to continue, the more difficult correction becomes and single binocular vision may be permanently lost.

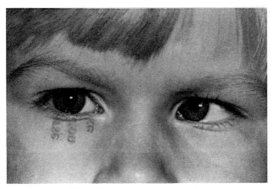

Fig. 7.2 *A convergent squint.*

There are generally no symptoms other than the physical deformity (Fig. 7.2) in the child presenting with concomitant squint. This may be noted by the parent, GP, health visitor or school doctor. Pseudo-squint, due to epicanthic folds giving the eyes a close-set appearance (Fig. 4.3), should be excluded.

Treatment of squint should commence as soon as possible as correction could be more difficult the longer it is left. A full examination of the eyes will be carried out to determine the cause and character of the squint. Four methods of treatment are available and are often used in combination.

Spectacles will be prescribed where necessary to correct any refractive errors noted by the ophthalmologist. *Occlusion* of the fixing eye may be useful to improve vision in an amblyopic eye. *Orthoptic treatment* is of great value in many cases and aims to restore or develop binocular function by special exercises. The child needs to be old enough to co-operate. *Surgery* is necessary in many cases and may need to be done in several stages. It aims to restore the visual axes to parallelism in all directions of gaze, and may be undertaken in children as young as one year.

A satisfactory cosmetic result can usually be obtained, but it is not always possible to restore binocular single vision and in some instances patients may experience double vision.

Incomitant squint or paralytic may occur at any age and is often the result of muscle or nerve damage following cerebrovascular disease, trauma, neoplasms or intracranial haemorrhage. An acquired incomitant squint may also be the first sign of disease of the central nervous system. It is essential to determine and, wherever possible, treat the underlying cause. Diplopia is often worst when the patient looks in the direction of the affected muscle and may lead to nausea and giddiness. Occlusion of one eye either with an occlusion patch or a Chevasse lens may be necessary to relieve the diplopia until corrective surgery is carried out if appropriate.

LATENT SQUINT (heterophoria)

Heterophoria can be regarded as a physiological condition. It may be present but only noticeable when the patient becomes debilitated or the stimulus to fusion is weak. Most patients are unaware of the presence of a latent squint. Correction of refractive errors and orthoptic exercises are usually the only forms of treatment necessary.

NURSING CONSIDERATIONS

- A nursing history and individual assessment of each child's needs should be undertaken with the help of his parents.
- Where possible, a parent should be encouraged to remain in residence and to participate fully in the child's care. If Ben's parents (see profile) had been counselled more thoroughly, their guilt feelings may have become apparent more quickly and steps taken to avoid the emotional trauma to both child and parents.
- When a parent is in residence, they should be made to feel welcome on the ward, and encouraged to participate as much as possible in caring for their child. They should not, however, be pushed into helping with every small detail, and the nursing staff should ensure that they receive adequate breaks, rest and food. Any new procedures which they are to learn, instilling eye drops, for example, should first be demonstrated by the nurse; the parent should then perform under supervision until competent to carry out the task alone. Individual assessment of each parent's capabilities will mean that they can be involved to their maximum potential.

- Clear information regarding preparation and operative procedures should be given to parents and child, in language which they can understand. It is important to remember that small children do not view events in the same way as adults and may react quite differently. They may be very excited at the prospect of a trip to theatre and an operation.
- Antibiotic eye drops are normally instilled three or four times a day both pre- and post-operatively. The means of instillation will depend on the age of the child. The very small child should be securely wrapped in a blanket and held on a couch by an assistant. The older child may co-operate better if teddy receives a drop first—it is usually best to lie the child down and ask him to put his hands under his bottom. The older child may sit during the procedure with his head well supported. In all cases, if at all possible, the nurse or parent should stand behind the child, separate the eyelids and instil the drops with the minimum of fuss.
- The eye is not usually padded following surgery, and so the nurse must ensure that the child does not rub his eye. He may wear his own spectacles.
- Prior to the child's discharge, normally one or two days after surgery, the nurse should be sure that the parent understands the orthoptic exercises and can instil the antibiotic drops.
- The parents should be assured that any redness of the eye will gradually subside. It should be emphasized that they may contact the hospital before the out-patient appointment (usually after one or two weeks) if they are worried.

FURTHER READING

Cashell, G.T.W. & Durran, I.M. (1974) *Handbook of Orthoptic Principles* 3rd Edn. Edinburgh: Churchill Livingstone.

8   The lacrimal apparatus

Tan Cheng Kim had been admitted to the ward previously with acute dacrocystitis and was now suffering from the condition again. She was a sad-looking lady of 50, whose only wish was to return to the Far East as soon as possible. The fact that she was in pain with a swollen face only made the situation worse. She spoke only in order to reply to questions and spent the first two days lying on her bed.

One evening, a Chinese nurse was allocated to the ward and was able to talk to Cheng Kim in her own language. It became apparent that she disliked Western food, but felt that she would be making a nuisance of herself if she asked her husband to bring in meals for her. She also felt that her accent made her English difficult to understand, and so she was reluctant to speak to the nurses too much as she felt they were busy and would not have time to try to understand her.

Fortunately, the situation was quickly resolved: Chinese food was brought in and the nurses made sure that they took time to sit and talk to Cheng Kim in quieter moments of the day. She remained a quiet and rather sad lady, but the rest of her stay on the ward was more relaxed and cheerful than it might otherwise have been.

The *lacrimal apparatus* is concerned with the production of tears and their drainage via the lacrimal duct into the inferior meatus of the nose. The apparatus consists of the lacrimal glands and their ducts, the puncta and canaliculi, the naso-lacrimal sac and duct and the accessory glands of Krause and Wolfring (Fig. 8.1).

The *lacrimal gland* is approximately the same size and shape as an almond and is lodged in its fossa (the lacrimal fossa) on the anterior and lateral part of the roof of the orbit. There is a flattened palpebral portion which may be seen through the conjunctiva in the outer part of the upper fornix when the eyelid is everted.

The gland consists of many pinhead-sized lobules which drain into fine lacrimal ducts. The 10–12 ducts drain tears into the outer part of the superior fornix.

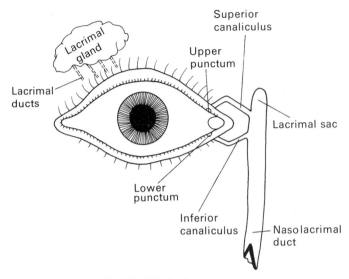

Fig. 8.1 *The lacrimal apparatus.*

Blood is supplied by the lacrimal artery, a branch of the ophthalmic, and drains via the lacrimal vein into the superior ophthalmic vein. Sympathetic nerve fibres control normal tear secretion but the lacrimal gland is also supplied by the Vth and VIIth cranial nerves.

THE LACRIMAL PASSAGES

The *lacrimal puncta* are located in the papillae at the nasal aspect of the upper and lower lid margins. They are kept patent (open) by the dense tissue surrounding them, and form the entrance to the L-shaped *canaliculi*. Each canaliculus extends vertically for about 2 mm before bending almost at a right angle to pass horizontally for 7–8 mm (see Fig. 8.1). The diameter of 0.5 mm can be tripled if necessary because of the elastic walls, and the canal may be straightened out over a probe. The upper and lower canaliculi join to form the common canaliculus before entering the lacrimal sac.

The *lacrimal sac* is dome-shaped and forms the upper portion of the naso-lacrimal duct. It lies in the lacrimal fossa in the anterior portion of the inner wall of the orbit.

The *naso-lacrimal duct* is 15 mm long and opens into the inferior meatus of the nose. The opening is usually slit-shaped and difficult to locate. The membranous lining of the duct is continuous with the nasal membranes, and infection passes readily between the two cavities. The rich blood supply of the duct means that engorgement of the membrane with consequent obstruction of the duct may occur. Sensory nerves are supplied from the Vth cranial nerve.

Tears are secreted at the rate of about 1 ml every 24 hours and act to:

(1) keep the cornea moist;
(2) prevent friction between the globe and eyelids;
(3) wash away foreign material; and
(4) counteract bacterial activity.

Tears are slightly alkaline and consist of 98.2% water, 1.3% sodium chloride, sodium bicarbonate and alkaline phosphate, and 0.5% protein in the form of lysozyme, an antibacterial enzyme. Tear production is minimal in the first weeks of life and decreases in old age.

Tears secreted by the lacrimal and accessory glands are swept across the eye by blinking. Some evaporate from the front of the eyeball and the remainder enter the puncti by capillary attraction. Horner's muscle contracts during blinking, creating a vacuum in the lacrimal sac which helps to draw the tears along the canaliculi into the sac. They then pass down the naso-lacrimal duct into the nose to be absorbed by the nasal mucosa.

The *tear film* consists of three layers:

(1) Superficial layer—composed of lipid from the meibomian glands. This prevents the rapid evaporation of tears.
(2) Middle layer—'tears' (see above).
(3) Deep layer—mucin from the goblet cells of the conjunctiva. This allows a smooth spread of tears by reducing the surface tension (allowing better 'wetting' of the cornea).

DISEASES OF THE LACRIMAL APPARATUS

Dry eye syndrome

Dry eye syndrome (keratoconjunctivitis sicca) has a wide variety of causes. Any disease that results in deficiency of any of the tear film components will result in dry painful eye and sometimes severe additional damage. It should be noted that tear production decreases with age with the absence of any other disease process.

Sjögren's syndrome is a form of keratoconjunctivitis sicca often associated with rheumatoid arthritis.

In most patients, the eye appears normal but they complain of burning or itching, a feeling that they have something in the eye but are unable to produce tears. There is often excessive mucous secretion and, on examination, the bulbar conjunctiva may look lack-lustre, oedematous and hyperaemic.

In order to assess the amount of tear production, *Schirmer's tear test* is often used. Performed without local anaesthetic, Schirmer's test will measure lacrimal gland function where secretory activity is stimulated by the irritating nature of the filter paper. The function of the accessory lacrimal glands may be estimated if the test is performed following the instillation of topical anaesthetics. A strip of filter paper is placed in the lower conjunctival sac and the patient is asked to keep both eyes closed for 5 minutes. At the end of this time the length of dampened paper is measured—anything less than 15 mm wetting is considered abnormal.

Dry eye is treated with artificial tears; a methylcellulose preparation is common and is effective as a corneal wetting agent. Tears that are produced should be preserved. Temporary blockage of the puncti and canaliculi may be achieved by inserting gelatine rods and if this is effective, permanent blockage may be achieved by cauterizing the puncti.

WATERY EYE

Watery eye may be due to:
(1) Lacrimal hypersecretion caused by pain, emotion or neurogenic factors such as a foreign body or excess light.
(2) An abnormal eyelid position which means that tears do not enter the punctum to drain.
(3) A lacrimal passage obstruction causing epiphora (a spilling over of tears). The stasis of tears which results commonly leads to infection—dacryocystitis.

DACRYOCYSTITIS

Congenital dacryocystitis occurs when there is an imperforate membrane at the base of the naso-lacrimal duct. There is often accompanying conjunctivitis, because normal drainage of tears is impeded and infection more likely to occur. The overlying skin may be swollen, red and tender. Pressure on the swelling may result in the discharge of mucopurulent matter through the punctum.

Treatment consists of regular massage over the lacrimal sac: this aims to create a vacuum which will open the naso-lacrimal membrane. Antibiotic drops may be prescribed where discharge is abundant, and these should be instilled three or four times daily for several months. The obstruction usually breaks down spontaneously but if it persists beyond about 12–18 months of age, probing of the lacrimal duct may be carried out under general anaesthetic. The child will normally be admitted and discharged on the same day.

Acquired dacryocystitis occurs in adults in whom there is partial or complete obstruction of the junction between the naso-lacrimal sac and the naso-lacrimal duct, causing the tears to pool and become infected. It is more common in females over 40 years of age and may be acute or chronic. Infection may ascend from the nasal mucosa and is commonly caused by staphylococcus, pneumococcus and haemophilus influenzae.

Acute dacryocystitis produces pain with swelling and redness of the overlying skin. The eyelids and submandibular lymph nodes may be swollen and the patient may be pyrexial. The patient may be admitted and treated with antibiotic eye drops after conjunctival swabs have been taken. Analgesia and systemic antibiotics will be prescribed and hot spoon bathing may help to relieve pain. Once the inflammation has subsided, dacryocysto-rhinostomy may be performed to prevent recurrence.

Chronic dacryocystitis is painless and non-inflamed. The patient notices persistent epiphora, especially on exposure to cold wind, dust and smoke. Pressure on the skin over the lacrimal sac will release pus or mucoid material through the punctum. Intra-ocular surgery is not generally performed in these patients, as the normal conjunctival sac is inundated with pathogens.

In the early stages, syringing (p. 33), passing a probe (p. 35), instilling antibiotic drops and regular massage over the lacrimal sac may effect a cure. For more persistent disease, dacryocystorhinostomy will be performed to establish free drainage from the sac in the nasal cavity by anastomosing the two and removing a portion of the intervening bone. A dacryocystogram (X-rays taken immediately following lacrimal sac washout with fluorescein) is usually requested prior to surgery.

CANALICULITIS

Inflammation of the canaliculi may occur following infection or an eyelash blocking the canaliculus, and may cause tearing and inflammation of the adjacent conjunctiva. Thick, 'cheesy', dirty yellow matter may be expressed from the red and swollen puncta. Curettage of the necrotic material in the affected canaliculus followed by irrigation is usually effective.

TRAUMA

Trauma may cause obstruction to the lacrimal passages if damage occurs in the region of the lower lid. Anastomosis of the torn canaliculi may be undertaken and in these cases fine polythene tubing will be inserted to maintain patency; it will normally be removed after three to six months.

NURSING CONSIDERATIONS

- Parents of those children suffering with congenital dacryocystitis will need to be taught to massage over the lacrimal sac area to clear the passages of pus prior to instilling antibiotic drops. The anatomy of the area should be simply explained with the aid of diagrams, and the nurse should ensure that they understand why and how to clear the ducts.
- Where probing of the lacrimal duct is necessary in infants with persistent dacryocystitis, as with any general anaesthetic, the nurse must ensure that the parents fully understand the necessity of withholding food and drink pre-operatively.

FOR PATIENTS UNDERGOING
DACRYOCYSTORHINOSTOMY

- These patients should be warned prior to surgery that a facial skin incision will be made. Although facial incisions usually heal well, the patient should be warned that scarring may result. This is particularly important if the patient is prone to keloid scarring. Any worries that the patient may have should be talked through and the use of cover-up make-up discussed if appropriate.

- In addition to the general preparation for general anaesthesia, some surgeons may request the patient's nose to be packed with ribbon gauze soaked in 4% cocaine with adrenaline 1 : 10 000, which acts to constrict the blood vessels and cause nasal mucosa shrinkage, thus reducing bleeding during operation which might obscure the view.

- Hypotensive drugs are sometimes used during surgery to make the blood flow more manageable in this highly vascular area. It is important that such patients have their blood pressure carefully monitored on their return to the ward until it returns to normal levels.

- A pressure dressing will be applied in theatre and should be observed for 'strike-through' (blood or exudate seeping through the dressing). If this occurs, additional padding should be applied; the dressing should not be removed for 24–48 hours.

- Daily syringing of the passages with isotonic saline normally begins on the third post-operative day unless silicone tubes have been inserted to maintain duct patency.

- For several days post-operatively, the patient should be discouraged from blowing his nose and from wearing spectacles since these may damage the fragile anastomosis. He will not be required to rest in bed, but his activity will be restricted if he relies on spectacles for normal sight—the nurse will need to be particularly sympathetic to the frustration that this will cause.

- *When nasal tubes are inserted* following repair of traumatic injuries or dacryocystorhinostomy, the patient should be warned that he may experience epiphora while they are in place.

- The tubes will be removed after three to five months, usually in the out-patient department. The patient should be seated comfortably with his head well supported. The front of the eye will be anaesthetized with Gutt. Benoxinate 0.4% and the tubes may then be eased gently upwards by manoeuvring them with forceps from inside the nostrils. The tubes may be cut with scissors close to the medial canthus while the patient looks laterally, and they are then drawn gently down the nose.

FURTHER READING

Lyle, T.K. & Cross, A.G. (1968) *May and Worth's Manual of Diseases of the Eye*. London: Baillière Tindall.

Martin-Doyle, J.L.C. (1975) *A Synopsis of Ophthalmology*. Bristol: John Wright.

Vaughan, D. & Asbury, T. (1974) *General Ophthalmology*, 7th Edn. Los Altos, California: Lange Medical Publications.

9 The sclera

Pat's knees were always painful—she worked as an office cleaner and felt that sore knees were a hazard of her job. For the past few days she had been even less comfortable because her eyes had become sore and red as well. She visited the local eye casualty on her way home from work one morning and thought it very strange when the doctor looked at her eyes, then asked about her knees and took a blood sample from her arm. Rheumatoid disease was diagnosed and explained to Pat, who now needs frequent treatment with steroid eye drops. She still has the symptoms of episcleritis but suffers less discomfort and is able to continue her work.

STRUCTURE OF THE SCLERA

The sclera is a dense, fibrous, almost entirely collagenous structure which forms the posterior five-sixths of the protective outer covering of the eye (the anterior sixth is cornea). The anterior visible portion of the sclera constitutes the 'white' of the eye. It may appear bluish in childhood as it is thin and the uvea shows through. The inner surface of the sclera is brown due to adherent suprachoroidal pigment and has marked grooves in which the ciliary nerves and vessels lie.

The sclera is about 1 mm thick and thins to about 0.3 mm anteriorly. At the site of the attachment of the optic nerve, the sclera becomes a thin sieve-like membrane, the *lamina cribosa*, through whose holes the retinal ganglion cell axons pass to form the optic nerve. The central retinal artery and vein also pass through the sclera at this point. When intra-ocular pressure is raised, as in glaucoma, the sclera 'gives' at this weakest point.

The outer surface of the sclera is covered by *Tenon's capsule* (fascia bulbi), a thin membrane, the posterior surface of which is in contact with the orbital fat.

There are three layers to the sclera:

(1) *The episclera*, the outermost layer of loose, vascular connective tissue and elastic tissue, connects the conjunctiva to the

sclera. It is, for the most part, continuous with Tenon's capsule.

(2) *The scleral stroma* consists mainly of bundles of collagen fibres, and gives the sclera its white colouring.

(3) *The lamina fuscia*, the innermost layer, is adjacent to the choroid which provides the melanocytes to give it its brown colouring.

Blood supply to the scleral stroma is via the episcleral and choroidal vascular network and the posterior ciliary arteries. Nerve supply is via the ciliary branches of the trigeminal nerve. Because of the rich nerve supply, scleral inflammation is usually painful.

FUNCTIONS OF THE SCLERA

(1) It maintains the shape and integrity of the eyeball by resisting intra-ocular pressure. In the adult, the sclera is inelastic, and forms a very effective anatomical protection for the contents of the eyeball, although it does stretch in response to raised pressure in infants.

(2) It forms an attachment for the extrinsic muscles of the eye.

DISEASES OF THE SCLERA

CONGENITAL ANOMALIES

These usually occur as colour alterations. Pigmentation may occur in diseases associated with iron or copper metabolism. Blue sclera are characteristically associated with deafness, bone fragility disease (osteogenesis imperfecta) and keratoglobus. Thinning of the sclera (staphyloma) may occur in congenital glaucoma.

INFLAMMATORY

Episcleritis

This relatively common condition affects women twice as frequently as men, and its peak incidence is between the ages of

30 and 40 years. It is usually unilateral, although it may occur subsequently in the other eye. The episcleral inflammation may be a manifestation of systemic disease; this is usually collagen disease, although *Herpes zoster*, tuberculosis and gout may be present.

The onset is sudden, and the patient presents with pricking pain, lacrimation, photophobia and an oedematous, red sclera.

Fifty per cent of the inflammations resolve spontaneously within three weeks. Intensive therapy with anti-inflammatory drops, often steroids, will be needed until the redness clears. Any underlying disease must be treated simultaneously.

Scleritis

This is a more serious and more painful condition which tends to be bilateral and recurrent. The onset is insidious, with generalized orbital aching turning to severe pain radiating to the frontal sinuses. Photophobia and visual disturbance are common. The complications can be severe (e.g. retinal detachment and treatment with anti-inflammatory drops should be commenced as soon as possible). Systemic corticosteroids or even (rarely) scleral graft may be necessary.

There is often an underlying systemic disease, which is collagen disease in 50% of cases.

TRAUMA

Chemical burns may destroy the collagen fibres, necessitating scleral and conjunctival grafting.

Laceration of the sclera invariably involves the underlying uveal coat and is most serious. Perforation of the sclera was common in road traffic accidents, although its incidence has been dramatically reduced with the compulsory wearing of seat-belts.

Contusion is most likely in the posterior part of the sclera and in the area adjacent to the canal of Schlemm. There is usually a history of blunt trauma or of a 'contrecoup' blow to the head.

NURSING CONSIDERATIONS

- Particular care must be taken when bathing the eyes of a patient with scleritis and in instilling medications. The sclera becomes thin and fragile and is easily damaged.
- Subconjunctival injections are never administered when scleritis is present, because pressure caused by the injected drug may rupture the diseased sclera.
- Scleritis is an extremely painful condition and the nurse should ensure that patients are given adequate effective analgesia.
- Long-term treatment with corticosteroids may result in scleral thinning, raised intra-ocular pressure and glaucoma in some patients, and the nurse should be careful to detect any changes at an early stage.
- The nurse's main role is one of supporting and guiding the patient in the management of their own treatment; for example, by ensuring that they can instil any eye drops prescribed.

FURTHER READING

Miller, S.J.H. (1984) *Parsons' Diseases of the Eye*, 17th Edn. Edinburgh: Churchill Livingstone.
Perkins, E.S., Hansell, P. & Marsh, R.J. (1986) *An Atlas of Diseases of the Eye*, 3rd Edn. Edinburgh: Churchill Livingstone.

10 The cornea

Alf Bell was 42 years old when he was admitted for a corneal graft. The corneal opacities were as a result of previous interstitial keratitis, a complication of measles in childhood. He had been married for four years and had a baby daughter whom he had never been able to see because of his corneal opacities. Although not obvious to a casual observer, the opacities in the pupillary regions of both eyes greatly reduced his visual acuity. Donor corneae became available and three days after the operation, his eyes were left undressed and he wore dark glasses. His wife and baby visited that afternoon and Alf wept with the joy of seeing his baby at last. Most of the other patients seemed suddenly to need to blow their noses.

STRUCTURE AND FUNCTION

The transparent tissue of the cornea covers the anterior one-sixth of the eye. It is about 11 cm in diameter and its curvature is slightly greater than that of the rest of the globe. The cornea and sclera are structurally continuous though separated by a slight furrow at the corneoscleral junction or limbus.

The smooth, transparent, curved structure of the cornea has a major role to play in vision. Light rays are refracted towards the lens by the cornea, which has a dioptic power of 40. This means that corneal injury can result in an impaired ability of light to pass through the structure and in loss of refractive accuracy.

The cornea is avascular, although the corneoscleral limbus is richly supplied. The corneal nerves are sensory branches of the ophthalmic division of the trigeminal nerve. The cornea is the most sensitive tissue of the body and stimulation of the nerve endings triggers pain, blinking and reflex tear production. Those patients with desensitized corneae, for example the unconscious or following *Herpes zoster* infections of the cornea, are extremely vulnerable to minor trauma and secondary infection.

The avascular cornea is nourished by the conjunctiva, which overlaps it anteriorly, and by aqueous humour at its posterior surface. Tears provide salts and protein, and oxygen is derived from the atmosphere.

The cornea consists of five distinct tissue layers (Fig. 10.1), the integrity of which is essential for transparency. The outer stratified pavement epithelium is continuous with the conjunctiva. It is extremely sensitive to touch but heals readily without scarring if injured. Bowman's membrane lies beneath the epithelium and normally adheres firmly to it. The membrane is resistant to injury and infection but does not regenerate if destroyed. This means

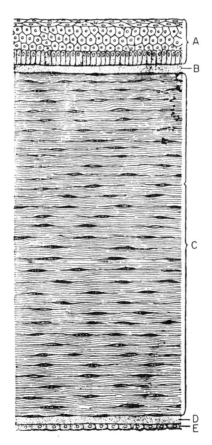

Fig. 10.1 *The histological appearance of the cornea. A, Epithelium; B, Bowman's membrane; C, stroma; D, Descemet's membrane; E, endothelium.*

that scar tissue will be formed by the process of healing. The stroma comprises about 90% of the total corneal thickness. It contains about 60 layers of flattened cells, laminae and numerous elastic fibres. Once destroyed, the architecture cannot be restored and opacity results. Descemet's membrane is a strong, structureless, resistant elastic membrane. It is resistant to chemical reagents and pathological processes but can regenerate if necessary. The deepest layer, the endothelium, consists of a single layer of flattened cells, which may be seen with the aid of a slit-lamp, the only place in the body where living endothelium can be viewed. It plays a vital role in controlling the amount of fluid in the cornea thus ensuring its transparency. Damage to the endothelial cells will result in an oedematous 'hazy' cornea which is less transparent than normal. The cells are unable to regenerate.

DISEASES OF THE CORNEA

The main symptoms of corneal disease are pain, iridescent vision (haloes) and reduced visual acuity.

CONGENITAL ANOMALIES

Megalocornea may be present at birth. The cornea continues to grow excessively and may be 15 mm in diameter in the adult: myopia tends to result. *Microcornea* usually occurs as a part of a generalized microphthalmos: hypermetropia may result.

DEGENERATIONS AND DYSTROPHIES

Arcus senilis is commonly seen in the elderly, in whom fatty degeneration produces a hazy grey ring about 2 mm wide just inside the limbus (Fig. 10.2). Arcus senilis causes no visual defect, there are no complications and no treatment is necessary.

Hereditary corneal dystrophies are rare and characterized by bilateral abnormal deposition of substances. There is alteration in the normal architecture of the cornea which may interfere with vision. The dystrophies usually manifest themselves during the

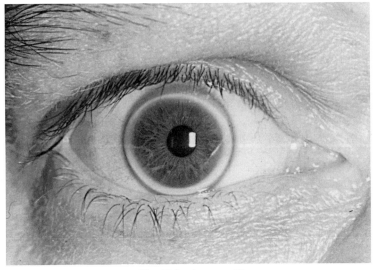

Fig. 10.2 *Arcus senilis.*

first two decades of life and may be stationary or progressive. They occur in the anatomical layers of the epithelium, stroma or endothelium.

CORNEAL INJURIES

Corneal foreign bodies account for the vast majority of ocular injuries that reach hospital and are more likely when dust, wind or smoke abound. The presence of a foreign particle will provoke vigorous blinking in an attempt to dislodge it. If this is successful the particle is washed way by the reflex flow of tears. Some particles may become trapped below the upper lid and must be removed by everting the lid. When foreign bodies become embedded in the cornea, good light and magnification may be necessary to remove them. Local anaesthetic drops should be instilled before removal either with a wisp of cotton wool or, for those particles that are more deeply embedded, with the point of a sharp needle. Mydriatic drops and antibiotic ointment will be instilled and a firm pad and bandage applied for 24 hours. The patient should be seen daily until any corneal damage has healed;

this may be determined by the instillation of fluorescein which will leave no green stain once healing is complete.

Corneal abrasion commonly follows minor trauma such as a foreign body. The corneal epithelium peels away from Bowman's membrane leaving a bare area that can be readily seen by instilling Gutt. Fluorescein 2% followed by normal saline, when the lesion will appear green. Local anaesthetic drops will relieve the sharp pain and the abrasion will heal quickly aided by instilling antibiotic ointment. Mydriatic drops and a firm pad and bandage will be necessary for large abrasions.

Perforating wounds of the cornea are often characterized by a collapsed anterior chamber and a gaping corneal wound. The iris and, more rarely, the lens and vitreous may prolapse. Treatment will depend on the site and extent of the wound and the presence of any complications. A careful history should be taken, and the retained intra-ocular foreign body excluded by radiography.

Simple perforating wounds are cleaned and sutured under anaesthetic and an air bubble may be injected into the anterior chamber in an attempt to prevent adhesions to the wound. Early removal of intra-ocular foreign bodies is essential if sight is to be retained. Many of these foreign bodies are metal fragments, such as when a hammer or chisel splinters during use, and may be removed with the aid of a magnet.

Sympathetic ophthalmitis is a complication which may occur following perforating corneal injury. An inflammatory response in the injured eye stimulates a uveitis in the uninjured or sympathetic eye. The usual treatment is removal of the injured eye before the sympathetic reaction becomes established.

Corneal burns may be caused by acids, alkalis, ultra-violet light or hot substances such as metal or plastic. Alkali burns should always be treated as an emergency since complications quickly arise. Prolonged irrigation with normal saline or sodium versonate is necessary to remove the alkali. Acid burns tend to be less serious since they coagulate the tissue protein, thus preventing deeper penetration. Tears help dilute acids but copious irrigation with normal saline or buffered phosphate is needed to ensure complete removal of the acid. People who are exposed to ultra-violet rays, such as in arc welding or sunlit snow, are likely to develop painful burns to the cornea about five to six hours after exposure unless protective goggles are worn. Treatment is with local anaesthetic drops and vasoconstrictors, e.g. Gutt. Adrenaline. Severe molten metal burns cause irreparable destruction of the corneal tissue. Less severe burns heal well, but often with residual scarring. Rodding of the fornices is necessary to prevent the formation of symblepharon.

KERATITIS

The normal healthy corneal epithelium is resistant to most organisms, but inflammation may be produced by bacteria, viruses or fungi. Corneal ulcers may be easily detected by staining the cornea with Gutt. Fluorescein 2%. The most common symptom of keratitis is photophobia, accompanied by pain and lacrimation. Inflammation will affect the transparency and curvature of the cornea, and defective vision results. Keratitis involving only the epithelium will heal in a few days without scarring, but opacity will result if the stroma is involved. Superficial opacity is termed a nebula, dense opacity a leucoma. Pus in the anterior chamber (hypopyon) may result from a particularly deep corneal ulcer.

Bacterial keratitis (corneal ulcer) is most commonly caused by a pneumococcal infection, although streptococcus and pseudomonas are also causative organisms. Pneumococcal ulcers tend to begin near the limbus as a grey, well circumscribed area and spread centrally. They usually follow corneal trauma. If untreated, the cornea may perforate and the eye may be lost. Pseudomonas keratitis spreads rapidly and may cause corneal perforation and permanent loss of vision within 48 hours. It often follows a minor corneal injury which has been examined with a *Pseudomonas*-contaminated fluorescein solution. Great care must therefore be taken to ensure that only sterile solutions are used.

The causative organism of bacterial keratitis should be isolated by taking a conjunctival swab so that appropriate antibiotics may be prescribed.

Viral keratitis ulcers are usually centrally placed and very superficial. The most common cause is the *Herpes simplex* virus. Intensive treatment with an antiviral agent such as acyclovir aims to halt the spread of the virus before debridement of the affected epithelium becomes necessary. The term *dendritic ulcer* refers to the appearance of *Herpes simplex* ulceration when the epithelial defects resemble a tree.

Epidemic keratoconjunctivitis is caused by an adenovirus transmitted from the upper respiratory tract. Incubation is usually seven to nine days and adults between 20 and 40 years are most commonly affected. Discharge and swelling are common additional symptoms and conjunctival haemorrhage may occur. There is no specific treatment, although antibiotic therapy will prevent secondary bacterial infection and antiviral drugs may be helpful.

In *Herpes zoster ophthalmicus*, infection with *Herpes zoster* virus may spread to the eyelids and cornea. Severe unilateral face pain precedes the eruption and rupture of vesicles. The eyelids become red, oedematous and painful, and fine dendritic lesions may occur on the cornea. The keratopathy may last for several months but usually heals with minimal scarring. Treatment consists of mydriatic and antiviral eye drops with analgesics for pain relief and antibiotics if the eye is sticky. This condition is dealt with in greater detail in Chapter 18.

Fungal keratitis is normally preceded by minor trauma such as a corneal foreign body or abrasion, often from a tree or other vegetable matter. A fluffy white spot appears and slowly spreads to involve the entire cornea. Treatment is with antifungal eye drops or ointment.

Where there has been a deeply eroding corneal ulcer, the cornea becomes thin and the underlying membranes balloon forward under intra-ocular pressure and are likely to rupture. Ballooning of Descemet's membrane is termed a *descemetocele*; if the deeper corneal lamellae are also involved it is termed a *keratocele*. Keratoplasty may be required later.

KERATOPLASTY (corneal graft)

Keratoplasty has been carried out in the UK since the 1930s and has become increasingly successful with the development of microsurgical techniques and fine instruments and sutures. The aim is to replace a scarred cornea, or part of cornea, with healthy tissue from another eye. Auto-graft, where the cornea is transplanted from one of the patient's eyes to the other, is rare, and most corneae are from cadavers or from eyes that have been enucleated for diseases not involving the cornea. The success of corneal grafting is largely due to the fact that the avascular cornea provides a bloodless barrier around the graft. Tissue typing and treatment wth steroid drugs also increase the success rate.

There are two types of keratoplasty:

(1) Lamellar or partial thickness graft, which is used to treat superficial opacities.
(2) Penetrating or full-thickness keratoplasty is more common. It involves opening the eye and thus a risk of introducing infection. There can also be problems with healing around the edges—the graft must be exactly flush with the existing cornea. Rejection is more likely with this type of graft. Both types of surgery are performed under general anaesthetic.

THE DONOR EYE

The Human Tissue Act 1953 allows an individual to bequeath his eyes for the purpose of corneal grafting. Cadaver eyes must be removed within ten hours of death by a doctor who, in practice, requires the consent of the next of kin. The eyes are stored in a refrigerator at 4°C for use as soon as possible, normally within 48 hours. The eyes should be free from glaucoma, malignant melanoma of the iris and corneal disease.

Many major cities in the UK now have eye banks established, and continuing research into freezing and storage techniques means that better use may be made of the available corneae.

PRE-OPERATIVE CARE

Patients are usually admitted 24–48 hours prior to surgery or may have been called in suddenly as donor material becomes available. Patients should always be warned that the donor cornea may prove unsuitable and the operation will have to be postponed. This inevitably leads to great disappointment, particularly in those who have been waiting for months or years, and the nurse will require a great deal of understanding, sympathy and tact in comforting and advising patients in these circumstances.

Pre-operative care includes the taking of conjunctival swabs for culture and sensitivity, the instillation of antibiotic drops and cutting the eyelashes of the affected eye (see Chapter 2). The pupil may be constricted with Gutt. Pilocarpine 2% prior to penetrating keratoplasty.

THE OPERATION

The operation is carried out in three stages:
(1) Preparation of donor material. The disc is cut under microscope control using a hollow trephine and is placed in sterile Ringers or saline solution. Where a lamellar graft is to be performed, the donor material may be removed after the affected portion of host cornea has been removed, so that the size can be matched accurately.
(2) The host eye is prepared by removing the diseased cornea either by 'shaving' for a lamellar graft, or with a trephine for a full-thickness graft.
(3) The donor cornea is placed onto the host eye and secured in place, usually using a continuous suture of 10.0 monofilament nylon. The opened anterior chamber is reformed with Ringers Lactate solution.

POST-OPERATIVE CARE

Once he has recovered from anaesthetic, the patient should be made comfortable with two or three pillows and asked not to lie on the affected side, or to make jerky movements with his head. His eye will remain padded and bandaged for 24–48 hours before being redressed. The nurse must be careful to explain the need for restricted movement in bed during this period.

The first dressing should be carried out in a dimly lit room if possible, and full explanation given to the patient prior to each stage of the procedure. The pad should be carefully removed, the eye swabbed gently and opened with great care. The nurse should then check that the graft is clear and secure with no lifting areas. The depth and clarity of the anterior chamber should be noted, as should the size and shape of the pupil and any corneal oedema.

A mydriatic may be given to dilate the pupil in an attempt to avoid adhesions between iris and cornea and antibiotic drops will be instilled. The eye will be redressed daily with paraffin gauze under the eyepad to lessen the risk of the patient acquiring a corneal abrasion from opening his eye. The new cornea will be without sensation and the patient will be unaware of any corneal abrasion he might sustain.

The patient will usually be mobilized gently after the first dressing and discharged after a week. He may require assistance at mealtimes if vision in the unoperated eye is poor. Stooping, lifting of heavy objects and jerking movements of the head must be avoided. The patient may find dark glasses helpful once the eye pad is removed. The eye should be examined carefully each day so that any signs of rejection of the graft may be detected early and preventive measures taken.

The patient will normally be discharged about seven days after surgery, having received careful instruction about the instillation of his medication. He should be told to return if he is at all worried and will normally be followed up as an out-patient. Sutures will be removed up to six months later, once healing is complete. This is generally done under local anaesthetic.

NURSING CONSIDERATIONS

- Many patients admitted for keratoplasty have little or no warning and little idea of what to expect. The nurse can help to relieve her patient's fears by explaining carefully what the procedure will be. Explanations may need to be repeated several times as an excited, fearful patient is unlikely to take in all that is said to him. He should be given as much opportunity as possible to ask any questions that he may have and the nurse should answer them as fully and accurately as possible.

- The operation will take place as soon as possible following the patient's admission to the ward, and this can lead to his feeling hurried and unable to express any fears and anxieties. The nursing staff, while preparing the patient as efficiently and quickly as possible, must endeavour to make him feel relaxed and allow him time to talk.

- Patients or their relatives may approach the ophthalmic nurse asking for information on how to donate their eyes after death. Some hospitals have a leaflet available on the subject, or an adviser who will talk to the enquirers. If neither of these is available, the nurse may refer the prospective donors to the Royal National Institute for the Blind who will supply further information on the subject. In recent years, with the increase in transplant surgery of all types, public awareness of the possibilities of organ donation has increased and many carry donor cards stating which organs they are willing to donate following their death.

- Prior to discharge following keratoplasty, the patient must be aware of the need to rest as much as possible and to avoid crowded environments and smoky atmospheres. The nurse's responsibility is to ensure that the patient understands why these measures are necessary since he is then more likely to co-operate. He will also need clear and careful instruction with regard to the continuing treatment for his eyes—such as the instillation of any medication. The nursing staff should ensure that the patient and/or his relatives are able to carry out the treatment effectively and understand how often it should be performed.

- Those patients who have undergone surgery for the removal of a foreign body will naturally be fearful, particularly in the immediate post-operative period, of losing their sight. The nurse will need to be reassuring and supportive but truthful in her dealings with these patients. The surgeon should warn the patient if there is a possibility that enucleation will be necessary, and the nurse should reinforce what has been said and allow the patient to express his fears, at the same time helping him to adjust to the possibility of being left with only one eye.

- An important part of the nurse's role in caring for patients following corneal injury and surgery is aimed at the prevention and control of infection. Because of the lack of blood vessels in the cornea, the immune system responds to infection slowly and by sending small blood vessels into the corneal tissue in order to combat pathogens. Once infection appears in the cornea, it is difficult to treat and scarring often results. Patients must be aware of potential hazards which may cause trauma and infection. Particular care must be taken in windy conditions to ensure that dust particles do not cause corneal abrasion. In the elderly, an adequate diet and good hygiene are important as marginal ulcers may occur if patients neglect their diet.

FURTHER READING

Miller, S.J.H. (1984) *Parsons' Diseases of the Eye*, 17th Edn. Edinburgh: Churchill Livingstone.

Newell, F.V. (1982) *Ophthalmology: Principles and Concepts*, 5th Edn. St Louis, Missouri: C.V. Mosby.

Trevor-Roper, P.D. (1974) *The Eye and its Disorders*, 3rd Edn. Oxford: Blackwell Scientific.

11 The uveal tract

Stewart complained of a sore eye and blurred vision when he got up one morning, so his mother ensured that he was in the eye casualty department within half an hour. Stewart was seen by a doctor who diagnosed acute anterior uveitis and arranged his admission to hospital to endeavour to establish a cause. Over the next few days many X-rays and blood tests were taken but all proved normal. Stewart's eye improved rapidly with treatment and he was soon ready for discharge. His mother was very reluctant to take him home as she was convinced something serious was wrong with Stewart. The factors underlying anterior uveitis were explained to her and she was praised for bringing Stewart to the hospital so quickly. Both Stewart and his mother were more relaxed when they left, knowing that they had taken the correct action and reassured that there was no serious problem on this occasion.

STRUCTURE AND FUNCTION

The uvea, or uveal tract, consisting of iris, ciliary body and choroid, forms the muscular and vascular coat of the eye.

The iris, the most anterior portion, is a thin circular disc perforated near its centre (usually slightly to the nasal side) by a circular aperture, the pupil, which varies in size in order to regulate the amount of light reaching the retina. The iris is attached at its periphery or root to the middle of the anterior surface of the ciliary body (Fig. 11.1); it is very thin at this point and frequently tears away (iridodialysis) as a result of contusion injuries. The pupillary margin rests on and is supported by the anterior surface of the lens. The iris divides the aqueous chamber into its anterior and posterior portions.

The iris consists of five layers:

(1) anterior endothelium;
(2) anterior limiting layer containing connective tissue fibres intertwined to form a dense matting;
(3) the stroma, loose connective tissue in which lie embedded the

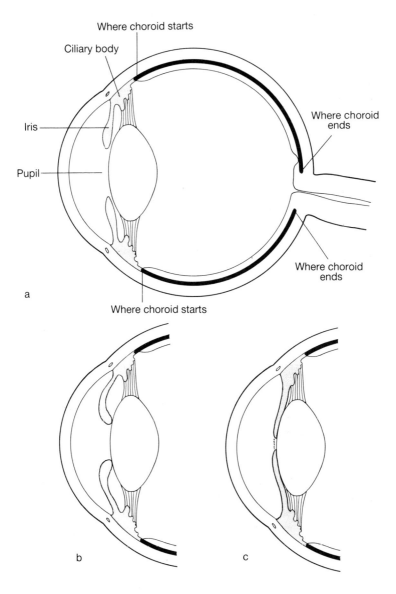

Fig. 11.1 *(a) The uveal tract. (b) Annular posterior synechia (occlusion of the pupil). (c) Total posterior synechia (occlusion of the pupil).*

sphincter pupillae muscle, the many blood vessels and nerves of the iris and the pigment cells;
(4) the posterior membrane of Bruch—a thin layer of muscle fibres, the dilator pupillae;
(5) posterior epithelium, which is highly pigmented and curls round the pupillary margin to form the black fringe of the pupil.

COLOUR OF THE IRIS

Most Caucasian babies are born with blue eyes because the stroma contains no pigment and the dark posterior epithelium is visible. With time, pigment is deposited in layers 2 and 3: little deposition will result in blue or grey eyes, large deposition will result in green or brown. In dark-skinned races, the stroma is pigmented at birth, while in albinism no pigment is deposited and visual defects result.

MUSCLES OF THE IRIS

There are two sets of smooth muscle fibres:

(1) The *sphincter pupillae muscle* is about 1 mm wide and forms a ring around the pupil. The muscle fibres are excited by bright light and contract, causing constriction of the pupil and consequent shielding of the retina. The pupil is also constricted in near reflexes and in sleep.
(2) The *dilator pupillae muscle* fibres radiate out from the pupillary margin. Constriction of these fibres results in dilation of the pupil, so that greater amounts of light enter the eye. This will occur in dim light and when the sympathetic nervous system is stimulated ('fright or flight').

THE CILIARY BODY

This forms a black ring connecting the choroid with the outer edge of the iris (Fig. 11.1). The epithelium of ciliary body is arranged in a series of ridges radiating inwards, the *ciliary processes*. These processes have a rich blood and nerve supply and produce and secrete aqueous into the posterior chamber by a process of ultrafiltration of blood. The greater part of the ciliary body is the *ciliary muscle*, supplied by the IIIrd cranial nerve (oculomotor). The muscle is arranged in two layers, the inner circular fibres or Muller's muscle and the outer longitudinal fibres or Bruch's muscle which are both utilized in the function of *accommodation*. The lens of the eye is attached to the ciliary body by the suspensory ligament, or zonule (Fig. 11.1), which relaxes when the ciliary muscle contracts. This results in decreased tension on the capsule of the lens which becomes more convex, allowing accurate focus on near objects.

THE CHOROID

The choroid is the highly vascular posterior portion of the uveal tract. It is a thin membrane extending from the optic disc to the ora serrata (the jagged line where the retina ends) at the ciliary body, and is placed between the retina and the sclera. The choroid is composed mainly of blood vessels arranged in three layers with the larger veins and arteries outside and the chorio-capillaries nearest the retina. Blood supply is from the short posterior ciliary arteries and drains via the four venae verticosae. These blood vessels supply the enormous nutritional requirements of the retina, particularly the metabolically active rod-and-cone layer. Heat is produced in the retina from the light striking it, and this is dissipated by the constant blood flow through the choroid.

The choroid contains many pigment cells, giving it its brown colouring, which reduce internal reflection of light and prevent leakage of light through the sclera. On rare occasions these pigment cells transform to produce choroidal melanoma, the most common malignant intra-ocular tumour.

DISEASES OF THE UVEAL TRACT

INFLAMMATORY

Anterior uveitis

Inflammation of any one component of the uveal tract usually spreads to the other two tissues but inflammation is generally more marked in the anterior portion. Patients usually present with pain which they describe as arising from inside the eyeball and which may keep them awake at night. Many experience photophobia which is unrelieved by wearing dark glasses, reflex lacrimation and a decrease in vision.

Examination will reveal engorgement of the episcleral blood vessels in the region of the ciliary body. The pupil becomes constricted and as the iris fills with exudate, pupil reaction becomes sluggish or non-existent. The iris may look blurred and may change in colour. Protein, fibrin and inflammatory cells appear in the aqueous which becomes translucent ('aqueous flare'). The iris exudate may spread to the back of the cornea and the front of the lens, and the iris may become adherent to these structures. The intra-ocular pressure tends to be lowered in the early stages but rises later with increased exudate viscosity.

In 90% of cases of anterior uveitis, no cause is ever found, but a wide range of systemic diseases can manifest themselves in this vascular layer of the eye: viruses, syphilis, tuberculosis, sarcoidosis, toxoplasmosis and ankylosing spondilitis have been implicated and should all be excluded, or treated if present.

Treatment of acute anterior uveitis is initially with topical mydriatics and steroids. If sufficiently severe, subconjunctival injection with these agents will be necessary. The eye is generally padded following subconjunctival injection; otherwise the eye is uncovered, but if photophobia develops dark glasses will give relief.

If left untreated, anterior uveitis may result in blindness or serious complications such as glaucoma, which occurs when normal aqueous drainage is inhibited because the trabecular meshwork is clogged with inflammatory exudate and large white cells. The 'sticky' iris can also adhere to the lens with disastrous results if left untreated.

Posterior uveitis (choroiditis)

Choroiditis is not seen on visual examination of the eye and is diagnosed with the aid of an ophthalmoscope. The patient usually presents with visual disturbance and mild photophobia, but little or no pain. They may complain of seeing floaters as debris appears in the vitreous. Often no cause is found (60% of cases), but viral infection, allergy, syphilis, tuberculosis, and collagen disease should all be excluded and treated if present.

Systemic steroids may need to be administered as local application is ineffective.

INJURY

Trauma causing bleeding from the iris will result in *hyphaema*, blood in the anterior chamber, a condition commonly seen in eye casualty departments. The injury may be a perforating one or, more commonly, blunt trauma such as a blow from a squash ball. Secondary bleeding may occur up to several days later, and patients are often admitted to hospital for rest and observation. Possible complications include glaucoma, iridodialysis and traumatic mydriasis (dilatation of the pupil due to the paralysis of the sphincter muscle of the iris—this may last for several weeks). Evacuation of the haematoma may be necessary, and the patient should be discouraged from taking strenuous exercise for several weeks to lessen the danger of a further bleed.

TUMOURS

Melanoma, both benign and malignant, may occur in the iris and the ciliary body. Benign tumours may be resected but enucleation is required for malignancy.

Choroidal malignant melanoma is the most common intra-ocular tumour. They most commonly arise from a pre-existing benign tumour and the malignant changes may be precipitated by injury or inflammation. As the choroid increases in volume, the retina becomes detached and there will be a loss of visual field in the area corresponding to the tumour.

Excision is sometimes possible in small tumours. Irradiation may also be used. Enucleation of the eye may be necessary if other means are inappropriate and where the eye is blind and painful.

NURSING CONSIDERATIONS

- Most patients with anterior uveitis will be managed as out-patients, and the ophthalmic nurse will play an important role in explaining the treatment and ensuring that the patient fully understands how to continue his therapy at home. Subcon-junctival injection can be particularly frightening for the patient, and a clear explanation from the nurse as to what to expect, i.e. a sensation of 'fullness' but not of pain, can go a long way towards inspiring confidence and ensuring the patient's co-operation.
- A wide range of blood tests and X-rays will be performed on patients with anterior uveitis, although an underlying cause for the inflammation is rarely found. The skilled ophthalmic nurse will assess her patients and tailor her explanations regarding these tests to suit their needs. She will require tact and ethical judgement if one of the tests is for syphilis and the patient wishes to know about the investigations in detail. Patients' questions should never be avoided or ignored and the ophthal-mic nurse should enlist help from a more senior member of staff if she feels unable to answer questions adequately.
- Many patients, having been subjected to a number of tests and investigations, find it difficult to accept that nothing serious is wrong. Again, the nurse will need great tact and patience in her explanations if the patient is not to feel foolish or misled. He should understand the importance of reporting any future symptoms quickly, and not be allowed to feel that he has wasted his own time and that of the hospital personnel.
- Patients with anterior uveitis or choroiditis generally feel well and become bored when hospitalized. To help relieve this nursing staff need to allow time for talking to and listening to the patient. Television and radio, books and free visiting can all help.

FURTHER READING

Sachsenweger, R. (1980) *Illustrated Handbook of Ophthalmology*. Bristol: John Wright.
Vaughan, D. & Asbury, T. (1974) *General Ophthalmology*, 7th Edn. Los Altos, California: Lange Medical Publications.
Wybar, K.C. & Kerr Muir, M. (1984) *Ophthalmology*, 3rd Edn. London: Baillière Tindall.

12 The lens

George Reed was a very fit and active 74-year-old whose great interest in life was athletics. He had worn spectacles for reading for many years but had no other problems with his eyesight until a few months before his admission. He had had to stop coaching athletics at the local boys' club because he felt as though he was constantly looking through a cloud. The haze seemed to be worse in bright light and he found it very distressing.

A diagnosis of bilateral, rapidly developing cataract was made. As the cataracts were affecting Mr Reed's life so much, he was admitted for lens extraction and intra-ocular lens implant to his right eye. When the dressing was removed, he was thrilled with the clarity of sight in the eye and wanted to know firstly, when the other eye could be done and secondly, what time did the football start on television.

STRUCTURE OF THE LENS

The lens is a transparent, avascular, biconvex body of crystalline appearance and is situated behind the iris and anterior to the vitreous body, where it is held in place by the suspensory ligament or zonule (see Figure 2.1). Its diameter is 9–10 mm and its thickness varies as the eye is focused on near or distant objects.

The anterior and posterior surfaces of the lens meet at the equator (Fig. 12.1). The posterior surface of the lens is slightly more convex than the anterior surface and lies in a shallow depression in the anterior vitreous face, the lenticular fossa. Nourishment is provided by the aqueous humour which constantly circulates across the anterior and posterior surface of the lens.

The lens consists of:

(1) The *capsule*, a transparent structureless, highly elastic envelope, which is thicker on the anterior surface and thickens further with age. When cut or ruptured its edges roll and curl outwards. The capsule keeps the lens in shape.

(2) The *anterior epithelium*, a single layer of cubical cells which

Lens

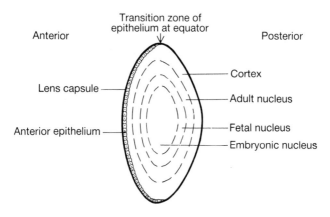

Fig. 12.1 *The lens.*

become columnar towards the equator and are eventually converted into lens fibres. There is no posterior epithelial layer.

(3) The *amorphous material*, a gel-like substance which binds together the lens fibres.

(4) The *lens fibres*, a series of long, prismatic six-sided bands, which lengthen and thin before breaking down. New lens fibres are laid down throughout life and as their central portions cannot be shed, the lens enlarges.

The lens changes colour with age from colourless to amber in old age, and while it gradually becomes larger it loses its ability to increase its convexity. It is held in place by the fine collagenous fibres of the suspensory ligament (zonule) which arise from the ciliary body and attach to the lens capsule on either side of its equator.

FUNCTION OF THE LENS

The lens's function is to transmit and refract light rays on to the retina. Its ability to increase its power of focus for near vision by altering its shape is termed accommodation.

When the ciliary muscle is relaxed, the suspensory ligament is taut and the lens is kept flattened by its taut capsule. When the eye looks at a near object, the ciliary muscle contracts and its diameter is reduced; the suspensory ligament is thus slackened and reduced tension on the lens capsule allows the lens to become more convex, shortening the focal length of light rays so that they can be focused on the retina (Fig. 12.2). The light is converted to light impulses and transmitted via the optic nerve to the brain for interpretation. Accommodation is always accompanied by pupillary constriction and convergence.

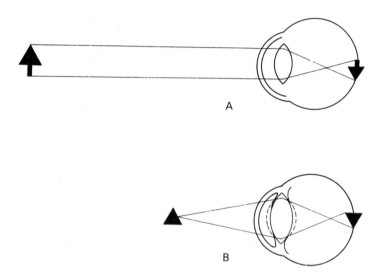

Fig. 12.2 *Refraction of rays of light. (A) From a distant object, more than 6 m away, rays are parallel. (B) From a near object, less than 6 m away, rays radiate from every point.*

ERRORS OF REFRACTION

Emmetropia, normal sight, occurs in the nearly spherical eye when vertical and transverse diameters are only 1 mm shorter than the anterior-posterior diameter (Fig. 12.3A).

Myopia, short sight, occurs when the anterior–posterior diameter is too long, and parallel light rays are brought to focus in front of the retina (Fig. 12.3D). A blurred image of distant

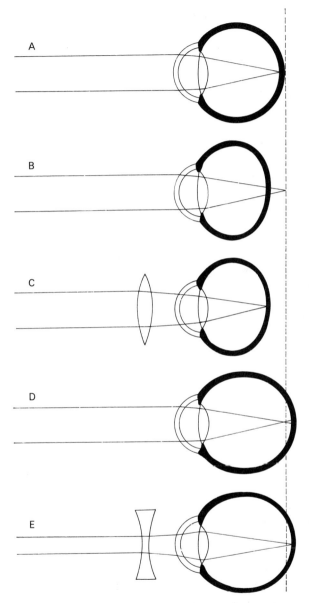

Fig. 12.3 *Errors of refraction. (A) A normal emmetropic eye – parallel rays are brought to focus on the retina. (B) A hypermetropic eye – the eyeball is too short and the rays are brought to focus behind the retina. (C) Hypermetropia is corrected by a convex converging lens. (D) A myopic eye – the eyeball is too long and the rays are brought to focus in front of the retina. (E) Myopia is corrected by a concave diverging lens.*

objects will result. There is a strong hereditary tendency to myopia though it is rarely congenital. It usually begins early in life and worsens through the growing years before improving in later life. In a few cases, retinal degeneration and detachment result (see Chapter 14). Myopia is corrected with a concave, diverging lens (Fig. 12.3E).

Hypermetropia, long sight, results from a short anterior-posterior diameter causing the image to be brought to focus behind the retina (Fig. 12.3 B). Near objects do not form a clear image on the retina. Vision is corrected with convex lenses which converge the light rays before they enter the eye (Fig. 12.3 C).

Astigmatism is a refractive error brought about by irregular curvature of the cornea. It is present to some degree in all eyes and is a congenital defect. It may also be acquired as a result of inflammation, injury or corneal surgery. It may be associated with myopia or hypermetropia. Treatment is by giving the lens added convexity or concavity in the appropriate meridian but vision will only improve after the lenses have been worn for some time.

Presbyopia develops from middle age as the lens loses its elasticity. Distant vision is unaffected but an inability to focus on near objects is a normal function of ageing. Ordinary print has to be held at arm's length or further in order to be read. Convex lenses are needed for reading and close work.

Refractive errors are corrected with spectacles or contact lenses, which have become increasingly popular in recent years.

CONTACT LENSES

Contact lenses are placed directly onto the outer surface of the eye and are available in three types; haptic or scleral lenses, microcorneal hard lenses, and soft lenses.

Contact lenses are most useful for correcting high refractive errors or for gross astigmatism which spectacles are unable to correct. Tinted lenses reduce glare in patients with albinism. Lenses may be used for cosmetic purposes in those patients with a disfigured eye following injury, those with a phthisical eye or with aniridia. Iris, sclera and pupil can all be painted on as appropriate.

Haptic or scleral lenses cover both cornea and sclera although refractive correction is provided only by the corneal portion. The lenses are bulky (see Fig. 12.4) but do not fall out readily Special lead-coated lenses have been developed to prevent eye damage during radiotherapy to the eyelids. Marked lenses can also be used to help pinpoint intra-ocular foreign bodies. The lenses require specialist fitting and are liable to exert pressure on the veins which drain aqueous, giving rise to an elevated intra-ocular pressure in patients with a narrow drainage angle (see Chapter 13).

Microcorneal hard lenses (Fig. 12.4) are the same size as the patient's cornea; they are less bulky, more comfortable and do not affect intra-ocular pressure. However, they fall out more easily and may cause corneal abrasions and limbal vascularization. The wearing time of both haptic and hard lenses must be gradually built up.

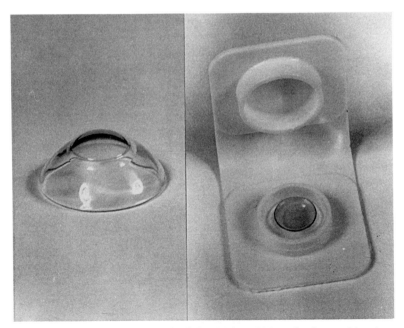

Fig. 12.4 *Contact lenses.* **Left,** *scleral (haptic) lens.* **Right,** *a hard corneal lens in a mailing case.*

Soft lenses are thin and gelatinous and have a water-absorbing property which makes them suitable only for those patients with an adequate tear flow. They are useful to protect the cornea when it is rendered vulnerable, e.g. by desensitization following keratoplasty or *Herpes zoster* infection. They will relieve the pain of bullous keratopathy by covering the exposed corneal nerve endings and act as splints to hold grafts in position. They are more comfortable than the hard types of lens and are readily adapted to by children following cataract extraction. Their life expectancy is, however, relatively short and they are more likely to become infected with organisms or contaminated from sprays. Soft lenses are more difficult to store and handle and must never be allowed to dry out (Fig. 12.5).

When receiving his contact lenses, the patient is taught how to care for them and how to insert (Fig. 12.6) and remove them. He will quickly develop his own techniques. Various solutions may be used to clean, rinse and store the lenses before insertion. Some

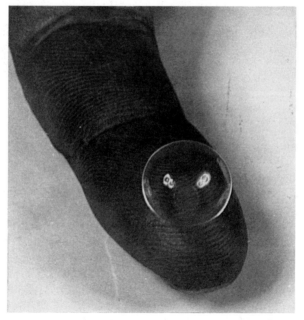

Fig. 12.5 *A soft contact lens balanced on a finger prior to insertion. The white marks are reflections of the camera flash.*

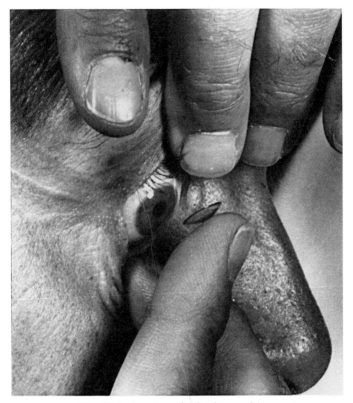

Fig. 12.6 *Insertion of a hard corneal lens.*

people find contact lenses extremely difficult to tolerate and many need to persist for several months before they feel really comfortable. Hard and soft lenses should not be worn during sleep, and the nurse must learn to check for contact lenses in injured patients, especially the unconscious, and be able to remove them.

There are several methods of removing contact lenses which involve manoeuvring one or both eyelids behind the lens and flipping it out into a waiting hand. Lenses can also be removed by holding the eye open and pulling the lens gently off using a special moistened rubber suction pad (Fig. 12.7). All nurses should familiarize themselves with this method of lens removal.

Once removed, hard lenses should be cleaned and may be stored dry, although they should not be banged about. Soft lenses

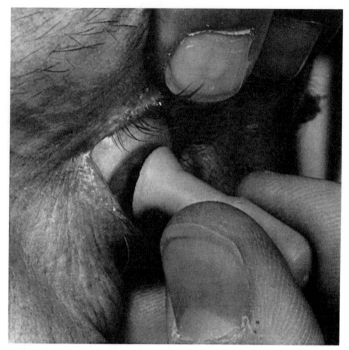

Fig. 12.7 *Removal of a scleral (haptic) lens using a sucker.*

should be cleaned with the appropriate solutions and stored in a container containing a sterile soaking solution. All contact lenses should be stored in special cases with separate compartments clearly marked for right and left lenses.

The prevention of corneal damage by infection or minor trauma is the major aim of management of patients who wear contact lenses. The nurse can play an important role in educating the patient regarding strict hygiene and good practices. She should also stress the importance of prompt treatment if any problems arise. Patients may be tempted to think that their lenses are simply uncomfortable for no apparent reason and be unaware of the insidious onset of corneal infection. The nurse should also warn any of her patients who are pregnant that their lenses may become uncomfortable, and they may need to revert to wearing spectacles until the pregnancy is over.

CATARACT

Because the lens is avascular it cannot support an inflammatory reaction and its only response to insult is to become opaque: a cataract is formed and the passage of light rays to the retina is interrupted.

Cataract is for the most part a disease of the elderly but may also be congenital or caused by trauma, metabolic disease or exposure to irradiation.

SENILE CATARACT

The lens tends to become opaque with age and by the age of 70 years, over 90% of the population shows some evidence of cataract, though visual impairment is often slight and progress negligible. The onset of the condition is gradual and the length of time before patients consult a doctor is extremely variable, depending to a large extent on their lifestyle and the importance to them of good vision.

Two types of senile cataract are distinguishable. *Nuclear* or *hard cataract* is an accentuation of the normal sclerosing process. The lens becomes cloudy, then yellowish and may eventually become brown or black. *Cortical* or *soft cataract* occurs when fluid collects in the lens and forces itself between the lens fibres. The lens has a cloudy appearance but actual opacities only occur when the lens proteins become denatured and coagulated.

When a patient presents, a diagnosis of cataract is easily made as the lens changes can be seen through an ophthalmoscope. It is important at this time to assess the patient's general health and to exclude any other causes of failing vision. Surgery will normally be undertaken when the patient can no longer see sufficiently well with either eye to continue his normal activities. The length of time this takes varies greatly from individual to individual.

CONGENITAL CATARACT

Some cataracts are present at birth, others occur in the early years of life as a result of congenitally determined defects. They may occur as a result of hereditary, nutritional or disease processes, perhaps the best known example being that of cataract in the infant whose mother contracted rubella during the first trimester of pregnancy. Cataracts may also be present in infants with Down's syndrome.

Visual acuity is difficult to assess in small children but, as a general rule, surgery will probably not be necessary if retinal blood vessels can be seen with an ophthalmoscope when the pupils are widely dilated. Nystagmus, retinal or choroidal abnormalities, microphthalmia and squint reduce the likelihood of good post-operative vision.

Binocular congenital cataracts which render the baby blind should be removed by needling or aspiration within a few months of birth, or earlier. If only one eye is affected, surgery may be delayed until the child is older—about five or six years—as long as vision is improved by spectacles. If the cataract is dense, light will not penetrate to the retina and the child will be amblyopic; surgery would not improve this and would therefore not be undertaken.

TRAUMATIC CATARACT

Any trauma which tears the lens capsule will allow aqueous to enter the lens and cause a local opacity. If the tear is large, most of the lens matter will be dissolved in the aqueous and an empty, wrinkled capsule sac will be left. The liberated lens matter may provoke an iritis or glaucoma.

Concussion cataract may occur after indirect trauma or after electric shocks, notably lightning, or the injudicious use of gamma- or X-rays. The lens capsule is intact and the opacity commonly remains localized to the posterior cortex in radiating fronds, the so-called 'sunflower cataract'.

METABOLIC CATARACT

These cataracts are related, directly or indirectly, to endocrine malfunction, diabetes mellitus and hypoparathyroidism being the two most common causes. They are bilateral and often develop rapidly.

True diabetic cataract is rarely seen today as diagnosis tends to be made early due to routine urinalysis tests and subsequent control of hyperglycaemia. Senile cataract tends to develop about 10 years earlier than usual in the diabetic patient.

TOXIC CATARACT

Corticosteroids systemically administered in high doses over long periods, notably to those patients with arthritis, may cause posterior subcapsular opacities in susceptible individuals.

SECONDARY CATARACT

Cataract may occur as a result of various intra-ocular diseases which interfere with lens metabolism; high myopia, retinal detachment, prolonged uveitis and intra-ocular tumours. They seldom merit removal.

RADIATION CATARACT

Cataracts may occur as a result of over-exposure to ionizing radiation or extreme industrial heat (they are found in glass-blowers and chain-makers). There is often an increase in the refractive power of the lens so that patients are able to read without their spectacles.

TREATMENT

Lens opacities, once present, are irreversible; the protein cannot be 'uncoagulated' and the only way to disperse them is to remove the lens. Similarly, there is no known method of preventing the progress of any naturally occurring cataract. During the period of decreasing vision, frequent and accurate refraction will allow vision to be maintained at the best possible level. In those patients with small opacities in the axial (central) areas of the lens, dilation of the pupil with drops such as mydrilate 1% may provide visual improvement by allowing them to see through the unaffected periphery of the lens.

Surgical treatment will normally be carried out when corrected vision is less than 6/18, but depends on the patient's own visual requirements. It may be much worse than this before surgery is undertaken in patients with systemic disease, where special risks are involved. Extraction is not justified if the patient cannot distinguish light and the direction from which it comes, as this implies gross retinal damage.

In the past, unilateral cataracts were not normally removed, as comfortable binocular vision was impossible with spectacles because of the dissimilarity of the two lenses. Full binocular vision is now possible either by contact lens or intra-ocular lens implant surgery.

Extraction of cataract may be achieved by removing the lens complete with capsule or by removing the capsule contents only.

Intracapsular lens extraction may be performed under local or general anaesthetic, and the lens removed, complete with capsule (see Fig. 12.8). Use of the proteolytic enzyme alphachymotripsin behind the iris a few minutes prior to lens removal helps to dissolve the zonular fibres supporting the lens, thus easing removal. A peripheral or sector iridectomy is normally performed to prevent post-operative glaucoma.

The advantage of intracapsular lens extraction is that there is no capsule remaining. This method is necessary if an iris lens clip implant is being inserted (Fig. 12.9), following lens extraction. There is, however, a very slight risk of vitreous loss with this method.

Extracapsular lens extraction: after the section has been made and peripheral iridectomy performed, a cystitome is used to make a series of incisions in the anterior capsule in the shape of a ring. The anterior capsule is then removed, followed by expression of the lens nucleus. Care is taken to ensure that all lens matter is removed and this may require irrigation and aspiration. The posterior lens capsule is not removed (Fig. 12.10).

This is the method of choice, particularly in young people and high myopes. It is the method used when a posterior capsular

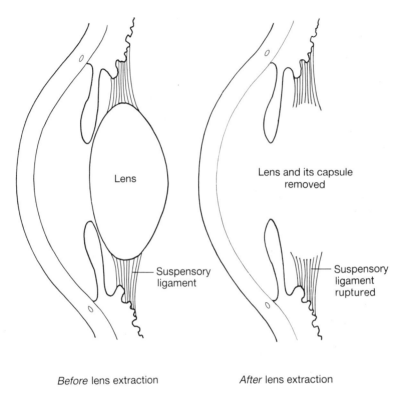

Before lens extraction   *After* lens extraction

Fig. 12.8 *Intracapsular lens extraction.*

lens implant is to be inserted. In this instance the anterior capsule must be removed apart from a small edge all round—microsurgery techniques have made this type of intricate surgery increasingly successful. A slight disadvantage of this method is that any lens fibres retained may cause 'after cataract' which may necessitate further surgery such as a capsulotomy (either by making an incision in the posterior capsule or by YAG (Yttrium–Aluminium–Garnet) laser) to provide clear vision.

Following removal of a cataract, a substitute lens must be offered to the patient. This may be either a spectacle lens, a contact lens or an intra-ocular lens. The thick lenses used in spectacles magnify objects up to 30% and hence make them appear closer than they are. The field of view is restricted because

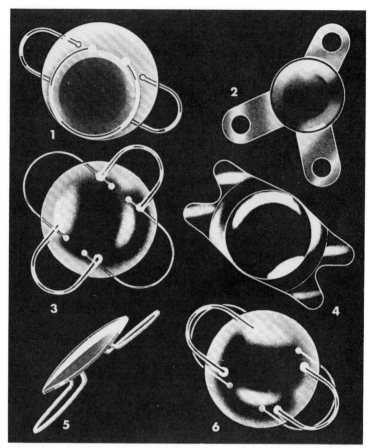

Fig. 12.9 *Intra-ocular lenses in current use. 1, The Worst two-loop implant; 2, the Rayner Pearce tripod posterior chamber lens; 3, iris lens clip; 4, the Rayner Choyce anterior chamber implant; 5, the iridocapsular lens, after Binkhorst; 6, the iris lens clip, after Binkhorst.*

the side field is distorted, and straight lines appear curved. Faces jump in and out of the blind area ('jack in the box' effect) during normal conversation and cause great annoyance. Cataract spectacles cannot be tolerated if the other eye has good vision.

Contact lenses magnify objects by only 6% but many elderly people (the majority of cataract patients) are unable to handle them adequately for them to be of use.

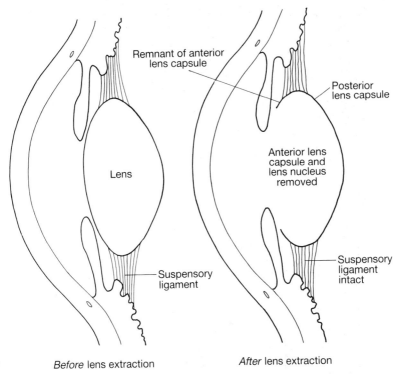

Before lens extraction   *After* lens extraction

Fig. 12.10 *Extracapsular lens extraction.*

Intra-ocular lenses may be implanted either at the time of surgery or some time afterwards. They give normal vision and are the corrective method of choice where possible.

NURSING CONSIDERATIONS

PRIOR TO PATIENT'S ADMISSION

- A major part of the nurse's role at this stage is helping to allay the anxiety of the patient waiting for cataract surgery. She should endeavour to ensure that he understands what has happened to his eye(s), and that nothing sinister is suspected. She may need to re-explain what the doctor has said if the patient has failed fully to understand. Some idea of the likely length of time before the patient is called for operation will also be helpful, since the patient will be more likely to cope with deteriorating vision if he knows that it will be improved in, say, three months.

- A nursing assessment may also be made at this stage so that the effects of deteriorating vision on the patient's normal daily activities may be estimated. Individual assessment is essential since there are such wide variations between patients. It may be possible to arrange for a patient to receive help at home if certain activities are severely restricted (home help, district nurse, meals on wheels, etc.). The nurse may also be able to advise on alternative activities and interests which will not be affected by failing eyesight.

PRE-OPERATIVE PERIOD

- The patient will usually be admitted a day or two before planned surgery in order to ensure that they are fit and medically prepared. At this stage the nurse's aim is to make them feel as relaxed as possible by welcoming and orientating them to the ward environment. It may be helpful to introduce them to a patient who has recently undergone successful surgery for cataract.
- A full nursing history will be taken and the patient's problems noted so that action can be taken to lessen or resolve them.
- Relief of her patient's anxieties and fears will again be an important part of the nurse's care. The patient may be worried by the thought of operation, at being in hospital, about his family at home and about what to expect following the operation. The nurse should assure herself that the patient understands what will be done in theatre and what he may expect on his return to the ward, particularly if he will be required to remain in a particular position for the first 24 hours. Any other likely procedures should also be briefly explained.
- Pre-operative nursing care will be as for all patients about to undergo surgery but, in addition, conjunctival cultures may be required, eyelashes may have to be trimmed or lacrimal sac

washout performed. The appropriate pupil may be dilated 30 minutes before surgery.

POST-OPERATIVE PERIOD

- When collecting the patient from the theatre complex, the nurse should ensure that he is fit to return to the ward and that she understands precisely what surgical procedures were performed and any specific instructions regarding the post-operative period.
- In the initial recovery period her aim is to avoid the potential problems of obstructed airway and shock following surgery. She should nurse the patient so that a clear airway is readily maintained and should regularly observe his condition, including recording pulse and blood pressure, until she is satisfied that he is fully conscious and no longer at risk.
- A secondary aim will be to minimize the risk of further damage to the eye either from trauma or through infection. The patient should not lie on the side of the operated eye, since this may cause a rise in pressure and heightens the risk of trauma from objects such as pillows. The patient may need to be reminded not to turn over many times in his semiconscious state. The eye will be padded and bandaged, but patients should be encouraged not to touch the dressing since this may cause trauma or introduce infection. The dressing should be observed for strike-through (staining from inside) and extra pads applied if this occurs, since a moist patch will provide an ideal entry channel for bacteria. The dressing should not be removed at this stage. Vomiting can damage the eye so the nurse should ensure that an anti-emetic is prescribed and administered if the patient feels nauseated or if opiate drugs are given (they are known to cause nausea and vomiting in some patients).
- Any pain or discomfort which the patient experiences may be relieved with a change in position or prescribed analgesics.
- A regular evaluation of the patient's needs will highlight any activities with which he requires assistance—perhaps with eating and drinking or with personal hygiene. Movement should be kept to a minimum for the first 24 hours and the nurse

should ensure that the patient has ready access to a call bell and knows how to use it.

- At the first dressing, usually 24 hours after surgery, the nurse should explain fully all that will be done in an attempt to allay the patient's natural fears. The eyelids will be bathed and the eyes examined for signs of discharge, swelling or bruising to the eyelids, conjunctival haemorrhage, injection or oedema. The cornea should be observed for clarity and the anterior chamber for depth and clarity. Ensure that there is no iris prolapse or leak around the wound and that the pupil is of normal size and shape with no lens matter present. Any pre-scribed treatment should be instilled; commonly antibiotic and steroid drops and a mydriatic unless an iris lens clip has been inserted. A clean pad with strapping, bandage or a shield will be applied. Prevention of infection is the nurse's aim at this dressing, and strict asepsis must be maintained.

- For most patients, sight will be vastly improved by the oper-ation, and the nurse will be able to share their joy when the dressing is removed for the first time.

- The patient may need further reminders of activities which may damage the eye such as bending down or jerking his head suddenly. These should be avoided, although the patient may sit up in a chair and walk to the toilet.

- The operated eye will be covered and, in many cataract patients, sight in the other eye will be poor. This may mean that they need help with many simple daily tasks which they would otherwise manage for themselves.

- Treatment and redressing of the eye will continue as prescribed. On the second or third day dark glasses or temporary corrective spectacles are usually supplied. The nurse should demonstrate to the patient how to put them on so that there is minimal risk of injuring the eyes (see Figure 12.11). She should not leave the patient with his spectacles until she is satisfied that he understands the importance of this method and is proficient at it. The eye will normally be padded overnight.

- Prior to his discharge home, usually about five days after surgery, the nurse should ensure that her patient will be able to manage his own treatment. He or his friends/relatives will need to be taught how to instil any necessary medications. He should understand any changes that may be necessary in his

(a)

(b)

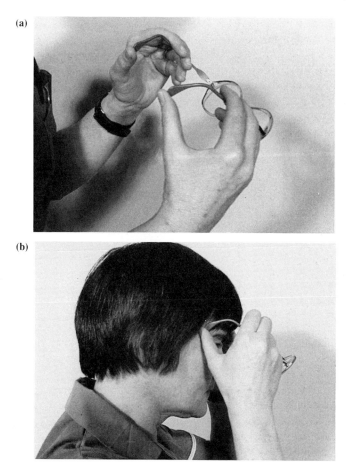

Fig. 12.11 *(a) A patient protects the ends of her glasses with thumbs, (b) Glasses are safely fitted without danger of the leg touching the eye.*

future lifestyle; sporting activities should be avoided, as should bending with the head down or lifting heavy objects. He may need help to wash his hair, for example, since he should not bend over forwards to do this. If necessary district nursing assistance or home help can be arranged.
- Follow-up will normally be about two weeks following discharge. The nurse should be sure that the patient knows when to return and has transport available.

FURTHER READING

Martin-Doyle, J.L.C. (1975) *A Synopsis of Ophthalmology*. Bristol: John Wright.
Miller, S.J.H. (1984) *Parsons' Diseases of the Eye*, 17th Edn. Edinburgh: Churchill Livingstone.
Stein, H.A. (1982) *Understanding Intraocular Lenses for Ophthalmic Nurses*. Canada: Pharmacia (Canada) Inc. and Intermedies Ophthalmic Products.

13 The aqueous humour

Betty Walton arrived in casualty during the evening insisting that she had glaucoma. She was a 45-year-old housewife who was normally fit and well, but for the past two days had experienced severe headaches and had vomited several times. Her left eye was red and painful and she could hardly see with it. She had seen her GP twice during this time and had been treated with topical antibiotics, but now she was desperate. When asked why she thought she had glaucoma, she said that her mother had experienced exactly the same symptoms at the same age and glaucoma had been diagnosed.

Aqueous humour is a clear, colourless fluid produced continually in the capillaries of the ciliary processes by a process of ultrafiltration. It is secreted into the posterior chamber and passes round the equator of the lens, behind the iris and via the pupil into the anterior chamber of the eye which it leaves through the trabecular meshwork. From there it flows into the canal of Schlemm and is drained by aqueous veins into the anterior ciliary and ophthalmic veins (Fig. 13.1).

Aqueous is 98.75% water and contains protein, glucose, ascorbic acid (vitamin C), lactic acid and a proteolytic enzyme. Its volume is about 0.3 ml and it is replaced approximately every 10 hours.

FUNCTIONS OF AQUEOUS

(1) The nourishment and oxygenation of the lens capsule, lens zonule, corneal endothelium and stroma, and the anterior vitreous.
(2) The maintenance of intra-ocular pressure.
(3) The refraction of light rays.
(4) Excretion: proteolyic enzymes break down inflammatory exudates and excrete them with the aqueous. Carbon dioxide is carried to the cornea for excretion from its surface.

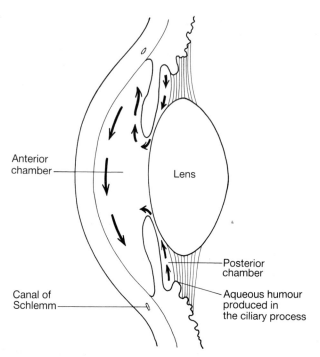

Fig. 13.1 *Circulation of aqueous. Aqueous passes through the pupil to circulate in the anterior chamber. It then passes through the trabecular meshwork into the canal of Schlemm.*

INTRA-OCULAR PRESSURE

Intra-ocular pressure is a measure of the resistance of the eye to external compression. It is maintained at a constant level between 10 and 20 mmHg, though with a diurnal variation of 3–5 mmHg. It depends on a perfect balance between inflow and outflow of the aqueous. Following trauma a lowering of intra-ocular pressure may lead to the condition of *hypotony* and may result in a shallow anterior chamber and serous choroidal detachment. If outflow is less than inflow, the condition of glaucoma exists and will cause pathological damage to the eye if untreated.

Intra-ocular pressure can be measured approximately by digital palpation of the eye (this is described in Chapter 3), which should feel like a 'ripe plum' if the pressure is normal. Precise measurement of the pressure requires the use of an applanation tonometer which measures the pressure needed to flatten a small area of the cornea. Some tonometers are used in conjunction with a slit lamp, and all are a potential source of cross-infection since they involve direct contact with the cornea. Careful cleaning of the tonometer heads is essential after each patient.

GLAUCOMA

Glaucoma is a disease characterized by raised intra-ocular pressure which impairs the blood supply to the optic nerve head, disrupting the visual field and, if untreated, destroying sight. The two main types of glaucoma are classified as *closed angle* and *open angle* (*chronic simple*) glaucoma. Medical treatment aims to maintain intra-ocular pressure within normal limits and so prevent loss of vision.

CLOSED ANGLE GLAUCOMA

In closed angle glaucoma, intra-ocular pressure is raised by an obstruction in the outflow of aqueous humour. It tends to occur in middle age as the lens thickens. It is usually bilateral and occurs more frequently in hypermetropes. The anterior chamber is shallow and the iris lies close to the drainage channels at the drainage angle. If the iris comes into apposition with the cornea, the drainage angle becomes closed off and a sudden rise in intra-ocular pressure (to perhaps 50–60 mmHg) ensues. This results in cloudy vision and a cornea containing too much fluid. An acute attack is most likely when the pupil is at the mid-dilation stage, as drainage from the posterior chamber to the anterior is minimal at this stage. The aqueous humour in the posterior chamber pushes the iris forward at its root and thus blocks the drainage angle. The use of mydriatics may precipitate an attack.

In the *prodromal stage* of closed angle glaucoma, attacks are intermittent and short-lived. They may be precipitated by stress and often occur in the evenings. Vision is blurred because of corneal oedema and the patient sees 'haloes'—coloured rings around lights—because corneal oedema results in diffraction of light. The eye feels painful, and if the patient is not treated with miotic drops or peripheral iridectomy, an acute attack is inevitable.

Acute glaucoma occurs when the drainage angle is closed off suddenly. The patient will complain of severe eye pain and head-ache, often accompanied by severe vomiting. He may experience lacrimation and photophobia in addition to a rapid, severe reduction in sight. On examination the eye will appear red and feel hard. The cornea is hazy due to oedema, and conjunctival chemosis and ciliary injection will be noted (see Fig. 13.2). The pupil will be semidilated, fixed and oval in shape, the anterior chamber shallow and the iris may look green, congested and dull.

Acute glaucoma is an ophthalmic emergency and one which the nurse in the casualty department should be able to recognize at once. Total loss of vision may occur if the pressure remains high for 24 hours. Patients will require hospital admission for treatment.

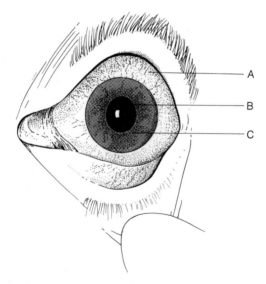

Fig. 13.2 *Acute closed angle glaucoma. A, the white of the eye is very red right to the junction with the cornea; B, the pupil is semi-dilated and slightly oval in shape; C, the cornea is slightly hazy.*

A carbonic anhydrase inhibitor such as acetazolamide 500 mg will be given intravenously to reduce the formation of aqueous. Treatment with miotic drops such as Gutt. Pilocarpine will constrict the pupil, drawing the iris away from the cornea, thus opening the drainage channels. Intravenous mannitol may be used if the intra-ocular pressure is insufficiently reduced—it acts to draw fluid from the eye by osmosis. Peripheral iridectomy or trabeculectomy will be performed once the intra-ocular pressure has been reduced.

OPEN ANGLE (CHRONIC SIMPLE) GLAUCOMA

Open angle glaucoma is a disease of middle age and develops insidiously over a period of time. It affects about 4% of the population over the age of 40 years but its course is often so slow that death precedes major sight loss. It is almost always bilateral, although more advanced in one eye.

Patients usually experience no symptoms until the disease is well advanced and visual field defects are large. Routine examination by an optician may reveal cupping of the optic disc and/or increased intra-ocular pressure before the patient has experienced any symptoms at all.

Intra-ocular pressure is usually raised, at least for part of the day, to about 30 mmHg or more. Cupping of the optic disc occurs because this area is the weakest of the intra-ocular structures and the least resistant to raised pressure (Fig. 13.3). The blood supply to the optic nerve is inadequate. Retinal blood vessels may be nipped at the lip of the optic disc predisposing to branch retinal vein occlusion.

Visual field defects occur slowly with small isolated scotomata above or below the blind spot. The scotoma develops a typical shape—an *arcuate scotoma*—which may be demonstrated using a perimeter (see Fig. 3.9). As the field loss progresses, the vision becomes restricted to a small central area, often no more than 10 degrees from the visual axis, in which full vision may persist.

It has been suggested that all persons over the age of 45 should be screened for glaucoma, but this is probably unrealistic. Since the disease has a hereditary tendency, however, screening of relatives of glaucoma sufferers is advised by many practitioners.

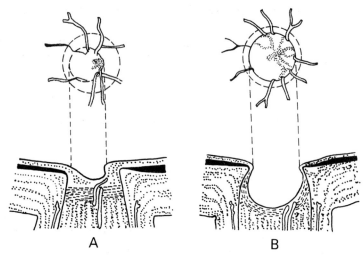

Fig. 13.3 *Cupping of the optic disc as seen on section of the nerve head and ophthalmoscopically. A, Physiological; B, pathological.*

INVESTIGATIONS

Various tests are available, many of them designed to provoke a rise in intra-ocular pressure when diagnosis is uncertain.

(1) *Assessment of intra-ocular pressure* should be undertaken over a period of 24 hours. If diurnal variation is greater than 4 mmHg or if the tension exceeds 30 mmHg at any time, chronic simple glaucoma may be present.

(2) *Water drinking test.* The patient is fasted from midnight and his intra-ocular pressure is recorded before breakfast time when he is asked to drink one litre of water within four minutes. This will lower the osmotic pressure of his blood and increase aqueous outflow from the eye. The intra-ocular pressure is then recorded at 15-minute intervals for an hour. A rise of more than 6 mmHg or a failure to return to normal pressure within an hour is diagnostic of underlying pathology.

(3) *Darkroom test.* Intra-ocular pressure is recorded before and after the patient has sat for one hour in a darkened room, as normal dilation of the pupil will cause some blockage of the

drainage angle. A rise of 5 mmHg or more is considered significant.

(4) The *mydriatic test* is an alternative to the darkroom test. A short acting mydriatic is used and again a pressure increase of 5 mmHg is significant.

These last two tests are not carried out on all patients.

(5) *Visual fields* are charted and visual acuity recorded.

TREATMENT

Medical treatment may be favoured in the first instance. With many patients, surgery is the treatment of choice. Visual fields and intra-ocular pressure should be recorded regularly and may involve admission of the patient. Full co-operation is essential if treatment is to be successful.

Pilocarpine eye drops 1–4% are instilled six-hourly. These act to constrict the ciliary body and open the trabecular meshwork, thus increasing the outflow of aqueous.

Beta-blockers, e.g. Gutt. Timoptol, inhibit aqueous production by the ciliary body, but their use is inadvisable for patients with heart failure, asthma or peripheral vascular disease. Carbonic anhydrase inhibitors, e.g. Diamox, or adrenaline analogues also may be used.

Surgery is performed if medical therapy is unsuccessful.

Trabeculectomy is the operation of choice, and allows the aqueous to drain out under the subconjunctival tissues. The aim is to prevent further visual field loss, and intra-ocular pressure should be lowered until blood flow to the optic nerve is adequate (this may necessitate a pressure as low as 10 mmHg).

SECONDARY GLAUCOMA

This type of glaucoma occurs when the intra-ocular pressure is raised because of previously existing eye disease, such as hyphaema, uveitis, lens swelling or dislocation. Topical steroids may cause secondary glaucoma in susceptible individuals.

The underlying cause should be treated wherever possible and acetazolamide may be used to lower intra-ocular pressure while treatment is undertaken. Surgery may be necessary if medical therapy is unsuccessful.

CONGENITAL GLAUCOMA

This is a familial disease and occurs when the anterior chamber is improperly formed in the fetus. Barkan's membrane remains and prevents aqueous from reaching the angle. Intra-ocular pressure is only mildly raised because the eye stretches to accommodate the additional fluid. The typical large eyes of babies with this disease (diameter greater than 12 mm) has given rise to the term '*buphthalmos*' (ox eye) to describe the disease. They also have hazy corneae.

Severely affected infants tend to bury their face in a pillow and scream, and the mother may notice photophobia and epiphora. The cornea is enlarged and hazy because of oedema, pupils are dilated and the sclera is thin and blue.

Congenital glaucoma is treated by performing a goniotomy or trabeculectomy to make an opening into the canal of Schlemm.

NURSING CONSIDERATIONS

- Great skill is required in the nursing of the patient with acute glaucoma. He will be in great pain as well as feeling extremely ill and will have the suddenness of emergency admission to hospital to accept. His fear of being blind is justified—full vision may not be recoverable.
- The nurse should explain his treatment to the patient, indicating what steps are being taken to control his pain and vomiting.
- The patient may have urgent domestic or professional problems which the nurse can help to resolve. Providing the patient with access to a telephone, or making necessary calls and passing on messages for him may do far more for increasing the patient's comfort than drugs alone.
- Eye drop therapy is necessary and the nurse must ensure that

strict standards of hygiene and safety are maintained throughout if infection is not to be introduced to the eye.

- Careful explanation of the aim of surgery will be necessary before the patient is taken to theatre; the nurse should satisfy herself that the patient understands that it is to prevent further visual field loss rather than to restore full vision.
- Extra caution will be needed when instilling eye drops in the post-operative period. Often a miotic and/or a beta-blocking agent will be prescribed for the unoperated eye, while the operated eye receives antibiotic and possibly mydriatic drops. It is essential that the nurse works on the side of the eye she is treating and that only the drops required for that eye are out on the trolley. Particular care should be taken in checking that the correct drops are being instilled.
- At the first dressing, usually after 24 hours, the depth of the anterior chamber should be accurately observed and any shallowness or flatness recorded and reported.
- The patient may require the nurse's assistance with activities such as getting to the toilet and may need help at mealtimes if vision in the unoperated eye is poor.
- Prior to discharge, great care must be taken in instructing the patient about his continued treatment, especially if there are different drops for each eye. If his vision is poor, it may be necessary to have easily distinguishable bottles.
- The nurse may help the patient come to terms with his future quality of life by ensuring, for example, that he understands the necessity of continuing his treatment after discharge, and the importance of long-term follow-up and monitoring.
- Where the patient is a child the nurse should spend time explaining the treatment to the parents and allow them time to ask questions and to discuss their child's future. They should be warned that the miotic drops will cause the pupil to constrict and that in poor light their child's vision may be impaired.
- For some children with congenital glaucoma, special schooling facilities may be appropriate and this may need to be organized; further details of the options available will be found in Chapter 19.

FURTHER READING

Henkind, P., Starita, R. & Tarrant, T. (artist) (1984) *Atlas of Glaucoma*. Fort Worth, Texas: Alcon Laboratories Inc. © Medical Dialogues Inc.

Miller, S.J.H. (1984) *Parsons' Diseases of the Eye,* 17th Edn. Edinburgh: Churchill Livingstone.

Sachsenweger, R. (1980) *Illustrated Handbook of Ophthalmology*. Bristol: John Wright.

14 The vitreous humour and the retina

Jennifer Lewis was 39 years old and a shopkeeper. She had closed her shop for the morning in order to attend the ophthalmic casualty department because she was so worried. The previous afternoon she had noticed flashing lights on the right side of her vision in her right eye. They stopped after a while and she continued working until her usual closing time. During the evening, while watching television, she noticed a black area in the vision of her right eye.

Jennifer's visual acuity was recorded soon after her arrival in the department and was satisfactory in both eyes, as was her intra-ocular pressure. Her pupils were then widely dilated and examination of the retina of her right eye showed a retinal detachment. The macular area was still attached (hence the normal visual acuity), and she was admitted to hospital at once for surgery later in the day to ensure that the macula remained attached.

THE VITREOUS HUMOUR

The vitreous humour is a colourless, transparent, gelatinous mass with a consistency a little firmer than raw egg white, which fills the posterior four-fifths of the globe between the lens and the retina (see Fig. 2.1). It is surrounded by an envelope, the hyaloid membrane, which lies in apposition to the retina but attached to it only at the ora serrata and the optic disc. If this membrane is ruptured by injury or surgery, vitreous will be lost.

Within the body of the vitreous, fine collagen fibres criss-cross to form a scaffolding. Some patients may complain of seeing small black 'floaters'—these are strands of collagen fibres which have broken away from the scaffold and are annoying but harmless, and this is a normal process. A sudden increase in the number of floaters or the additional symptom of seeing 'flashing lights' may indicate vitreous detachment or haemorrhage or retinal detachment and warrants investigation.

The vitreous has no blood supply but is nourished by the blood vessels of the retina, choroid and ciliary body.

If the vitreous gel shrinks and there is an abnormal adhesion of the vitreous to the retina, there is greater resistance and as the vitreous detaches it will tear a hole in the retina. Fluid is then able to pass through the hole, separating the nerve layers of the retina from the pigment epithelium which supplies its nourishment.

THE RETINA

The retina is the innermost layer of the eye and is part of the central nervous system, being an expansion of the optic nerve. It is a fine, delicate transparent membrane and is only visible in the living eye by virtue of the layer of blood vessels within it. The retina is thickest at the optic disc (1 mm) and thins to 0.5 mm at its outer extremity—the ora serrata. The retina lies between the hyaloid membrane of the vitreous and the choroid. The inner surface of the retina has a 'yellow spot' or macula lutea about 1.5 mm in diameter; this is the area of most distinct vision. Slightly below and to the nasal side is the optic disc which appears white and slightly raised; it is where the optic nerve enters and is composed entirely of nerve fibres which are not sensitive to light—the 'blind spot'.

The complex structure of the retina is shown in Fig. 14.1. The light-sensitive area is the layer of rods and cones, so called because of the shapes of the cells. There are about 125 million rod cells which are responsible for twilight vision and register black, white and grey impressions. They are the sole means of sight in dim light and contain the photochemical substance *rhodopsin* or visual purple, composed of vitamin A and the protein opsin. Rhodopsin breaks down as it absorbs low-intensity light rays and this releases energy to trigger off nerve impulses for transmission to the brain. Resynthesization of rhodopsin requires the presence of vitamin A and complete darkness—night blindness is a symptom of severe vitamin A deficiency.

The cone cells are confined to the central regions of the retina and are responsible for daylight vision and colour discrimination. They are particularly densely packed in the fovea centralis area

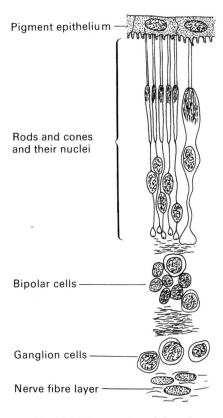

Pigment epithelium

Rods and cones
and their nuclei

Bipolar cells

Ganglion cells

Nerve fibre layer

Fig. 14.1   *Cross-section of the retina.*

of the macula, the area of fine visual discrimination. Particular cells discriminate particular colours and they are not equally distributed; the largest reception area is for blue, followed by red, yellow and green.

When light strikes the photoreceptors (rods and cones) of the retina, a photochemical reaction takes place which releases energy to trigger off a nerve impulse. The impulses pass to the bipolar nerve cell layer where they are organized into a meaningful pattern and relayed via the ganglion cell layer to the deeper nerve fibre layer. The axons of these nerve fibres become continuous with the optic nerve and transmit the impulses via the visual pathway to the visual centre in the occipital cortex.

DARK–LIGHT ADAPTATION

Adaptation to sudden darkness is a gradual process brought about by the increased sensitivity of the rods as the result of resynthesization of rhodopsin and by the dilation of the pupil which allows more of the available light to fall onto the retina. Sudden dazzling light following a period in gloomier surroundings also requires time for adjustment. Rhodopsin is bleached and the rod cells become less sensitive, while the pupils constrict and allow less light to enter the eye.

The retina's metabolic requirements are met by a dual blood supply; the pigment epithelium and the rods and cones are nourished by the choriocapillaries and the remaining inner layers by the central retinal artery.

A portion of the retina can be viewed through an ophthalmoscope. The macula appears as a small oval area devoid of blood vessels and vessels may be seen leaving the retina at the optic disc (Fig. 14.2). A number of retinal abnormalities may be seen by direct vision in this way, and every ophthalmic nurse should familiarize herself with the use of an ophthalmoscope. Retinal disorders present either with gradual and long-standing visual loss or with sudden, painless loss of vision in an apparently normal eye.

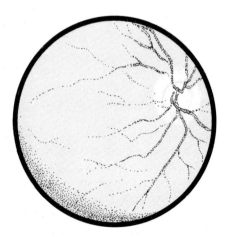

Fig. 14.2 *The normal fundus.*

RETINAL DISORDERS

RETINAL DETACHMENT

This disorder is more accurately called retinal separation, as the layer of rods and cones is separated from the pigment epithelium by tissue fluid. The retinal layers lie in apposition but are only attached at the ora serrata (outer edge) and at the optic disc, so that if the layers become separated for any reason, fluid from the vitreous will seep into the subretinal space. Since the retinal layers are nourished by the choriocapillaries, any separated areas will become ischaemic.

Patients may not notice any symptoms at first but may complain of flashing lights or spots in front of the eyes. Painless visual field loss may be experienced as though a curtain is spreading across the eye. The process may take only days or may go on for months before the eye is totally blind.

Primary detachment occurs when a hole in the neural layer allows accumulation of fluid between the neural and pigment epithelial layers—the retina floats off. Causes include high myopia, shrinkage or loss of vitreous humour and trauma, either blunt or penetrating.

Secondary detachment occurs when the retina is either pushed off the pigment layer, for example, by an intra-ocular tumour or choroidal haemorrhage, or when the retina is pulled off the underlying layers, e.g. when scar formation follows vitreous haemorrhage.

On examination, the area of retinal detachment appears grey with dark vessels crossing it. There are often crescentic folds in the retina, ballooning towards the vitreous (Fig. 14.3). Holes may be visible in the affected retina (Fig. 14.4).

The aim of treatment is to replace the retina in its original position. Prognosis will depend on the cause, the length of time the retina has been detached and the area involved. Surgery will aim to seal any tears in the retina, apply local pressure with a plomb and drain subretinal fluid.

Tears in the retina may be sealed by the application of intense cold ($-80°C$) using a retinal cryoprobe, which causes freeze burns resulting in adhesions between the choroid and retina.

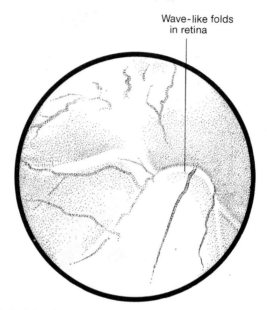

Fig. 14.3 *Retinal detachment. The detachment appears like a wave; the detachment area is slightly grey in colour.*

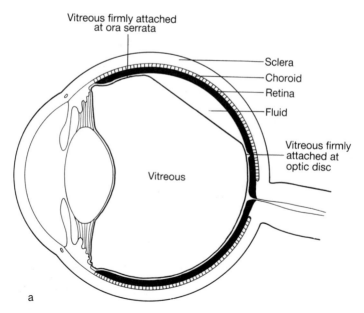

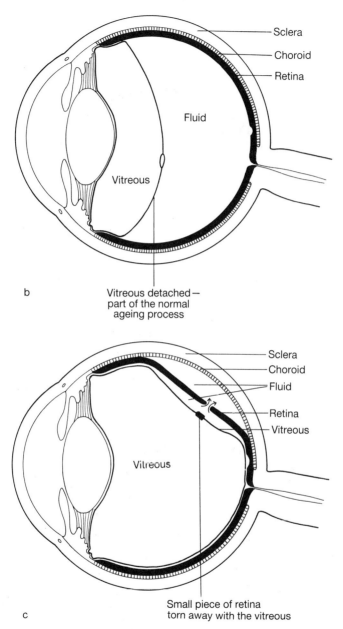

Sclera

Choroid

Retina

Fluid

Vitreous

b

Vitreous detached—
part of the normal
ageing process

Sclera

Choroid

Fluid

Retina

Vitreous

Vitreous

c

Small piece of retina
torn away with the vitreous

Fig. 14.4 *(a) Mechanism of retinal detachment. (b) Vitreous detached at the optic disc; this patient will complain of floaters like spiders. (c) A hole in the retina allows fluid to separate the retina from the choroid; the patient will complain of flashing lights.*

Local pressure may be applied externally by placing a silicone plomb on the surface of the sclera and covering it with conjunctiva to cause a local indentation, thus pushing the sclera, so causing the retinal pigment epithelium to come into contact with the retina again (Fig. 14.5).

Subretinal fluid may be drained through a hole in the sclera or may be allowed to absorb spontaneously once the retinal tear is sealed.

Where there is a tear but no detachment, the bond is strengthened by photocoagulation.

CONGENITAL AND DEVELOPMENTAL

Retinitis pigmentosa

This genetically determined degenerative disease usually has its onset between six and twelve years of age. Mainly the rods but also the cones degenerate and the retina develops a typical bone corpuscle pigmentary change. The condition is usually bilateral and the first complaint is often of night blindness. This is followed by a gradual progressive constriction of the peripheral visual fields and eventually blurred vision. Examination with an ophthalmoscope will reveal narrowed arterioles, pale yellow optic discs and pigment deposits throughout the retina, especially in the mid-periphery (see Fig. 14.6). Most sufferers have only tunnel vision by the age of 50 or 60 years, and have difficulty moving about in strange places, particularly in poor light, although most of them retain their reading vision until death. No treatment is available.

Senile macular degeneration

This progressive condition is the most common cause of blindness in the UK. Patients usually notice a gradual deterioration in vision with objects appearing smaller than usual and colours altered. This is followed by a central haziness or greyness and eventually by a blind area in the central field of vision. The macular area is the most vulnerable to degeneration, and its breakdown results in inability to identify faces, read fine print or discern colour correctly. Peripheral vision persists and sufferers are able to get

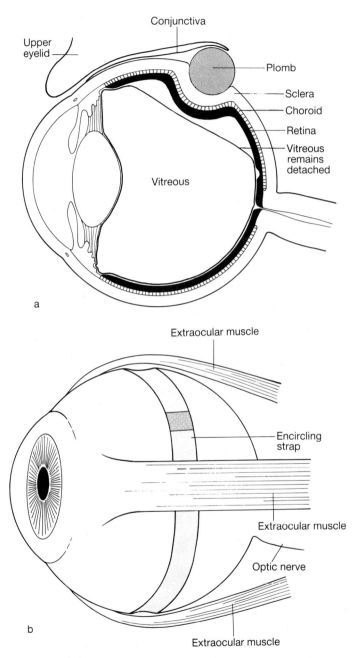

Fig. 14.5 *Retinal detachment surgery: (a) application of plomb; (b) attachment of encircling strap.*

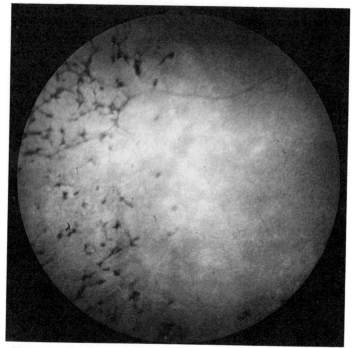

Fig. 14.6 *Retinitis pigmentosa, showing the peripheral 'bone corpuscles'.*

about. Senile macular degeneration is usually bilateral though more advanced in one eye.

Laser photocoagulation may be helpful, but is by no means a satisfactory cure. Patients may obtain benefit from the use of low visual aids, and may wish to register as partially sighted or blind.

VASCULAR DISORDERS

Central retinal vein occlusion (Fig. 14.7)

Patients may experience sudden loss of vision, but visual loss over a period of several hours is more common. The veins become thick and tortuous and multiple haemorrhages occur.

The condition usually improves spontaneously, although the formation of new blood vessels may block the drainage angle and cause a secondary glaucoma (rubeotic glaucoma). Any underlying cause such as hypertension should be treated.

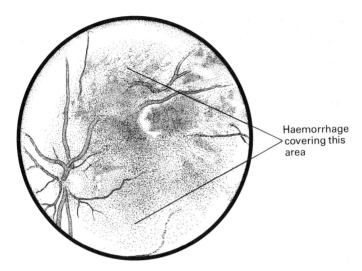

Fig. 14.7 *Thrombosis of a branch retinal vein.*

Haemorrhage covering this area

Central retinal artery occlusion

The central retinal artery supplies the central portion of the retina and its occlusion will result in sudden blindness. The main cause of the disorder is emboli from atherosclerotic plaques in the carotid arteries in the elderly, or valvular heart disease in the young. On examination, the retina looks pale and swollen and emboli may occasionally be seen within the retinal arterioles (Fig. 14.8).

Unfortunately, the condition is usually irreversible by the time the patient is seen, as the retina dies within a few minutes when deprived of blood. Vigorous massage of the globe may dislodge the clot and paracentesis (tapping) of the anterior chamber will be performed to lower intra-ocular pressure, causing the blood vessels to dilate and the clot to pass through.

RETINOBLASTOMA

Retinoblastoma is a malignant tumour arising most commonly from the inner nuclear layer of the retina. It is hereditary in many cases and may be present at birth. In about 30% of cases, the tumours are bilateral, though generally far more advanced in one

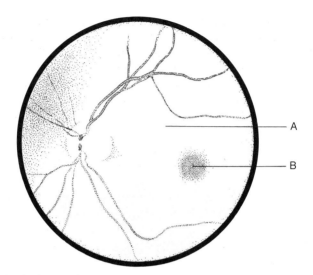

Fig. 14.8 *Occlusion of the central retinal artery. A, the fundus is pale instead of pink; B, there is a cherry-red spot at the macula.*

eye. The tumour grows either into the vitreous or into the subretinal space causing extensive retinal detachment. Left untreated, the tumour will fill the whole vitreous space, eventually causing glaucoma and rupturing through the sclera anteriorly to form a fungating mass. Spread is either to the orbital bones or via the optic nerve to the brain.

In those children in whom there is no suspicion of retinoblastoma, the tumour is usually advanced before it is diagnosed. A whitish mass may be noticed behind the pupil—'cat's eye pupil'. A very careful family history will be taken to attempt to ascertain a hereditary tendency and the parents' fundi should be examined for any signs of regressed retinoblastoma.

Treatment for advanced retinoblastoma is enucleation of the eye, taking as long a section of the optic nerve as possible. Where retinoblastoma is bilateral, the less affected eye will be treated by radiotherapy if possible in an attempt to retain some sight. If tumours in both eyes are advanced, bilateral enucleation will be undertaken, since irradiation of an advanced tumour would almost certainly result in destruction of the eye. Irradiation by means of a cobalt plaque attached to the sclera may be possible for small tumours, and light coagulation is occasionally sufficient.

The parents of children with retinoblastoma will require a great deal of counselling and help with regard to the future of their child, who may be severely visually handicapped or blind following treatment (see Chapter 19). Genetic counselling will also be offered, particularly in those instances where the condition is thought to be hereditary. Parents may require specialist help to enable them to deal with the feelings of anger, guilt and helplessness they may feel.

The child himself will require counselling when he reaches a suitable age since he may well pass on the condition to his own children.

Following surgery, the child will require admission to hospital every 8–12 weeks for careful examination under general anaesthetic to detect any signs of recurrence of the tumour. As he becomes older, examination may be done without anaesthetic and less frequently.

RETINOPATHY

A number of systemic diseases, including diabetes, hypertension, renal disease, atherosclerosis and toxaemia of pregnancy cause retinal disturbances. These will be dealt with in Chapter 18.

NURSING CONSIDERATIONS

• Patients who are to undergo surgery to repair a *retinal detachment* are often admitted to the ward a day or two prior to surgery and encouraged to rest in bed. Depending on the area of the detachment, it may be necessary to nurse the patient in a specific position with the separated area at the lowest point of the eye. This may mean that the patient is in an uncomfortable position; for example, on his left side with the foot of the bed elevated if the tear is in the upper, outer quadrant of the left eye. It is important that the nurse makes clear to her patient the reason for such action; namely so that the retina can settle and fluid beneath the tear can be reabsorbed, thus avoiding extension of the retinal detachment.

- Whenever possible, nursing the patient at rest in bed should be avoided because of the many problems this can cause. The patient may be allowed to sit upright in a chair, or may be positioned leaning on a pillow on a secure table in front of him. If the patient's movements are restricted he should be taught, and encouraged to carry out, deep breathing and leg exercises. The nurse may need to consult and co-operate with the physiotherapist in these instances.
- The pupils of both eyes will be widely dilated so that good views of the retina may be obtained through an indirect ophthalmoscope.
- The inability to read can be a source of great frustration for some patients, and the nurse should take all possible steps to ensure that her patient's boredom is alleviated. Radios, talking books, visits from relatives and friends who may read newspapers or books to the patient can all help, and the nurse should make herself available to talk to her patients as often as possible.
- Following surgery, the patient may be required to rest in a particular position to allow internal tampenad of the tear so that the tear and the air is at the highest point of the eye, particularly if gas or air have been injected into the vitreous.
- Dark glasses will be offered for comfort when the eye is uncovered.
- Mydriatic eye drops, steroids and antibiotics will normally be prescribed for the patient following surgery. He may also require a simple analgesic.
- Complications which may arise following surgery include bruising and swelling of the eyelids, glaucoma, hypotony with choroidal detachment and anterior segment ischaemia. The nurse should look for signs of these so that treatment can begin early. Later, the plomb may extrude through the conjunctiva and require removal or it may become infected. Redetachment can also occur, necessitating further surgical intervention.
- Prior to discharge, normally after 7–10 days, the nurse should ensure that the patient understands and is able to instil his prescribed medication. He should also be advised to avoid stooping, lifting heavy objects or playing sport for several weeks. Those who are normally engaged in heavy manual work

may need assistance in arranging a lighter alternative—the social worker or DHSS Disablement Resettlement Officer may need to be contacted. Home circumstances should be assessed and any local authority services which may be beneficial, e.g. a home help or Meals on Wheels, may be arranged before the patient is discharged.

- A follow-up appointment will normally be made for two weeks following discharge and then as thought necessary by the surgeon. Most patients who have suffered retinal separation will be reviewed every 6–12 months.

- The nurse who is involved in caring for patients with retinoblastoma will need to be aware of her potentials and limitations, particularly when dealing with distraught parents. It is often the nurse to whom the parents turn and she should develop her skills of listening and ensure that she makes time to spend with such families. She should accept that she may find the situation personally distressing and be prepared to cope with her own emotions, seeking help and support from her colleagues where necessary.

- False reassurance should never be offered to such parents and the nursing staff may need to arrange several meetings between the parents and senior medical staff until the prognosis is properly accepted and understood.

- Parents may take out their frustration and aggression on members of the nursing staff. This will often be in the form of verbal abuse, and the nurse may need great patience and tact in dealing with such situations. She must also know when the parents require specialist help to deal with their feelings and make necessary arrangements.

- Parents will need to be taught to administer their child's treatment as soon as possible, and should handle an artificial eye prior to surgery if appropriate. Many parents find the removal of an artificial eye, cleaning of the eye socket and reinsertion of the prosthesis most distasteful to watch, and are extremely fearful at the prospect of having to perform the tasks themselves. The nurse will need skill to encourage the parents to co-operate and assist, and will need to stress how important it is that the child should not be aware of the parent's distaste and distress.

FURTHER READING

Miller, S.J.H. (1984) *Parsons' Diseases of the Eye*, 17th Edn. Edinburgh: Churchill Livingstone.

Perkins, E.S., Hansell, P. & Marsh, R.J. (1986) *An Atlas of Diseases of the Eye*, 3rd Edn. Edinburgh: Churchill Livingstone.

15 Traumatic injury

Ted was an 18-year-old who went joy-riding in someone else's car and had a crash. He sustained severe penetrating laceration right across the cornea of the right eye, and laceration to both upper and lower eyelids plus the bridge of his nose. Such injuries would not have occurred had he been wearing a seat belt.

Since the wearing of seat belts became compulsory, injuries such as those sustained by Ted have dropped dramatically.

Ted was uncooperative his entire stay in hospital. He never mixed with the other patients; nor would he speak to the staff except when he had to.

Ted's injuries healed following surgery, but he had a scar across the middle of the cornea which affected his vision and would require grafting later. The eyelids also healed, but would require further surgery later.

Traumatic injury to the eye may occur as the result of blunt trauma, penetration of the eye by a sharp object or damage caused by irritant chemicals. The eye alone may be affected, or it may be that injury to the eye is only one of many, perhaps serious, injuries to various parts of the body.

BLUNT TRAUMA

The eye is well protected from injury by the orbital bones (see Chapter 5), but is most vulnerable at its temporal side.

Bruising commonly occurs following blunt trauma. The swelling and bruising (ecchimosis) of the eyelids normally reabsorbs spontaneously. Conjunctival bruising will cause subconjunctival haemorrhage; again it will resolve spontaneously without permanent damage. Blunt trauma flattens the eye, increasing the diameter and stretching the sutures.

Bleeding may occur into the anterior chamber (hyphaema) as the result of blunt trauma, and this is clearly visible with the naked eye (Fig. 15.1). This will stop and absorb spontaneously

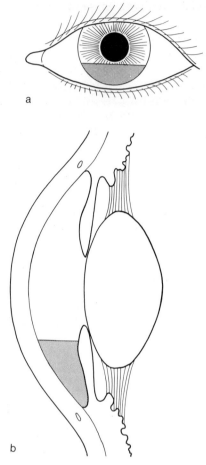

Fig. 15.1 *Hyphaema. (a) Blood in the anterior chamber obscures the iris. (b) Blood in the drainage angle can block the trabecular meshwork.*

through the iris and the canal of Schlemm. Haemorrhage into the vitreous will occur if the retinal blood vessels are damaged. Although it will clear if left untreated, there is the possibility that vitreous organization will form and lead to retinal detachment. Bleeding into the sheath of the optic nerve may cause permanent loss of vision if the nerve is compressed and its blood supply impaired. Immediate drainage of the orbit may on occasions be indicated.

Blunt trauma may cause a number of structures within the eye to *rupture or tear*. The cornea will give at its weakest point, at the limbus, and the sclera either around the canal of Schlemm or at the optic nerve. The iris will tear away from its root (iridodialysis); the choroid usually ruptures on the macular side of the optic disc and will not heal. The retina may also tear, sometimes as the result of long-standing oedema from previous trauma. In rare instances, the optic nerve may be torn from the sclera. Visual impairment will depend on the location and extent of the damage, but the patient will require admission for surgical repair.

Blowout fracture of the orbital floor (Fig. 15.2) may occur if intraorbital pressure is sufficiently raised as the result of a severe blow. This is detected on X-ray, and is most apparent when the

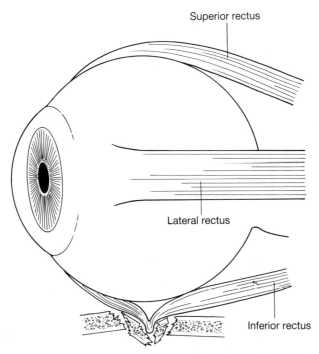

Superior rectus

Lateral rectus

Inferior rectus

Fig. 15.2 *Fracture of the orbital floor, with inferior rectus incarcerated in the fracture.*

inferior rectus muscle prolapses into the fracture. The patient often complains of double vision and especially on elevation. Surgical emphysema may occur around the orbit if he blows his nose. Once any haematoma and emphysema has subsided they may be assessed for possible surgical repair with a silastic implant. This is not always successful, and the patient may experience continued diplopia and require further surgery to repair a squint.

Opacity of the lens will result from damage to it, which may be accompanied by dislocation into the anterior chamber or into the vitreous. Surgical intervention will almost certainly be necessary if the lens dislocates into the anterior chamber or behind the iris, as it can block off the drainage angle by pushing the iris forward.

PENETRATING INJURY

This category of ophthalmic trauma may include anything from a very fine linear laceration of the cornea to a deeply penetrating injury through any part of the eyeball, causing gross disorganization of the eyeball contents. Small particles travelling at high velocity, such as metal fragments from a hammer or chisel, are most likely to penetrate as the patient does not have time to take evasive action.

Corneal foreign bodies and abrasions constitute about 25% of all ocular injuries and are generally very painful. The eye will water profusely and the patient will blink rapidly to try to remove the offending object. The eye should be anaesthetized before irrigation is commenced. If the foreign body will not wash off it may be brushed off with a damp cotton wool bud or lifted off with a needle. However it is achieved, it is important that the foreign body is removed in its entirety. The eye will be padded and bandaged following the instillation of an antibiotic to prevent the eyelids from causing further damage. A short-acting mydriatic will prevent ciliary spasm and so reduce the pain. Corneal epithelium is quick to regenerate.

Conjunctival foreign bodies frequently lodge on the upper tarsal conjunctiva and may not be removed simply by irrigation. Eversion of the upper lid and removal of the object with a cotton bud may be necessary. A large laceration will require suturing but small conjunctival abrasions will heal spontaneously.

Intra-ocular foreign bodies often lead to complications, notably infection, particularly if they are not removed immediately after the injury. If the history of the injury in any way suggests the possibility of a retained intra-ocular foreign body, X-rays will be ordered. A corneal contact lens with metallic markers may be used to help to locate the foreign body accurately. A tiny fragment may have left only a minute corneal tear, the edges of which have anastomosed leaving the eye looking normal, so that history of the incident is important in assessing the likely damage.

Some intra-ocular foreign bodies, e.g. coal and glass, are inert and may be left if there is no medical reason to remove them. Metal fragments will be removed, as will plant material such as fragments of twig, since these readily cause infections and destructive reactions. Foreign bodies lodged in the lens do not require removal as they become encapsulated.

Topical subconjunctival and systemic antibiotics will be used following surgical removal of a foreign body in order to minimize the chance of infection. Another possible complication is *sympathetic ophthalmitis* which may develop as a whole uveal tract inflammation in the uninjured eye. This complication is most unlikely if the injured eye is removed within a few days following injury. Severely damaged eyes with little chance of good visual recovery are often removed to prevent this serious complication.

BURNS

Burns to the eye may be caused by heat (or extreme cold) or by electricity, ionizing radiation or chemicals. In many instances, particularly in domestic accidents, the eyelashes, lids and brows are burned but the eyes are protected by the reflex closure of the lids and the evasive action of the patient. Such superficial injuries will heal quickly due to the excellent vascular supply to the face.

THERMAL BURNS

Thermal burns are often the result of industrial accident and are most commonly caused by hot metals. The depth and severity of the burn is usually directly proportional to the heat of the causative substance. Metals with a relatively low melting point, e.g. lead, zinc and tin, cool quickly and cause less severe burns than substances such as glass, iron, steel and slag (iron impurities mixed with limestone from the furnace), all of which have a melting point above 1000°C. In general, the burns are less severe than might be expected as the metal remains in contact with the eye for only a short time before falling off. Slag, however, has a rough surface and tends to adhere to the eye, producing a more severe burn.

The heat involved sterilizes the site at the time of injury but care must be taken to avoid secondary infection by the use of antibiotic drops. The resultant injuries usually heal well, but leave scars which cause opacities of the cornea and fibrous healing bands of the conjunctiva and the skin of the eyelids. Rodding of the fornices will be necessary if there is a threat of symblepharon formation. Entropion and ectropion from eyelids scarring are not easily prevented and will need surgical repair once the burns have healed.

ELECTRICAL BURNS

Domestic power currents rarely cause burn damage to the eyes, but the greater voltage carried in high-tension cables over or under ground or the enormous voltage of lightning will certainly be sufficient. Flash burns will cause injury to the eyelids and facial hair and skin, but current passing through the body causes far greater damage and often causes cataracts, partial or complete. Bilateral cataracts will mean that the patient requires surgery to restore his vision, but this may be delayed for a considerable time by the injuries to other parts of the body which may be extensive and severe.

RADIATION BURNS

Burns may be caused by infra-red, ultra-violet, X- and γ-rays.

Infra-red radiation is transmitted to the retina via the cornea and lens, and may cause chorioretinitis if the temperature of the tissues is increased sufficiently. *Eclipse blindness* is a form of infra-red burn caused by looking at the sun's eclipse with the naked eye. Burn damage to the retina is permanent and the patient will suffer impaired visual acuity, often seeing a black spot in the centre of his field of vision. The lens will absorb some of the rays and cataract may develop. Protective goggles should be worn by people whose employment exposes them to infra-red light, e.g. chain-makers and glass-blowers, and persons wishing to view an eclipse of the sun should only look at the projected image reflected, for example, in water.

Ultra-violet rays cause burns to the cornea and conjunctiva and occur in arc welders, those exposed to sunlit snowfields and those who expose themselves unwisely to sun lamps. Symptoms occur five to six hours after exposure and include intense pain, lacrimation and blepharospasm. Staining the corneal epithelium with fluorescein will demonstrate damage. Prevention may be achieved by the wearing of goggles or glasses designed to absorb the harmful rays. Although the condition is self-limiting and no permanent damage results, symptoms will be treated with local anaesthetics and antibiotics and oral analgesics.

X- and γ-rays often used in hospitals will cause cataract in exposed eyes. They also cause vascular changes in the iris and ciliary body and may result in glaucoma. Prevention is by the use of suitable lead shields, often in the form of contact lenses, to protect the eyes. If cataract develops, it may need to be removed.

CHEMICAL BURNS

Chemical burns may be caused by acids and alkalis.

The acids which most commonly cause burns to the eyes are sulphuric, hydrochloric, nitric and acetic. They destroy the tissues of the cornea and conjunctiva by corneal perforation and cicatrization (scar formation). Scarring of the cornea affects its transparency and reduces visual acuity. The skin, eyelids and sclera may also be affected and symblepharon, entropion and ectropion may result. The neutralizing solution for acids is Buffered Phosphate.

Burn injuries from alkalis are often more serious than those from acids, as they continue to release hydroxyl ions into the tissues which penetrate the sclera, so causing full-thickness burns.

Soda, potash, ammonia and lime (quicklime or slaked lime) are the commonest causes of alkaline burns. Lime burns tend to be the most serious because it is deposited as insoluble calcium salts. Lime is found in many commonly used agents—plaster, whitewash, gardening and farming products. The chelating agent for alkalis is sodium versonate.

The initial treatment of chemical burns is to irrigate the eye without delay. Running tap water is adequate until the patient can be moved to a casualty department, where irrigation will continue with copious amounts of fluid (either the specific neutralizing solution or, if this is not available, isotonic saline) for at least 15 minutes. If possible, local anaesthetic drops should be instilled prior to irrigation as it is important that the eye, including the fornices, is thoroughly cleansed. Rodding of the fornices will discourage symblepharon formation and any further treatment will depend on the extent of the damage. Dark glasses may help to relieve the pain caused by bright sunlight, and analgesics and antibiotics will be prescribed if there is corneal involvement.

NURSING CONSIDERATIONS

- A brief history-taking should precede any treatment to the eyes, except in the case of severe injury where immediate action is clearly necessary. The nurse must avoid wasting time by asking unnecessary questions, but should try to find out the cause of the accident and the order in which events occurred, with approximate times if possible. It may be appropriate to ask whether protective goggles were being worn and whether this type of injury has occurred previously at his place of work.
- Appropriate emergency treatment should be undertaken without delay, particularly where the patient has sustained chemical burns or where a foreign body on the conjunctiva or cornea is suspected.
- Some eye injuries are very apparent, for example hyphaema, and the nurse must be careful not to miss more serious but less obvious ophthalmic injury.
- Once emergency treatment has been carried out, a full ophthalmic nursing assessment may be carried out—this is described in Chapter 3.

- Many patients with traumatic eye injuries will have sustained injury to other parts of the body. It is essential that the nurse looks at her patient as a whole person, and does not miss important signs such as the onset of shock or deterioration due to an unrecognized head injury. Any patient who has been involved in a road traffic accident or who has a history of head injury should be examined thoroughly on arrival and regular recordings of his vital signs should be made. There is no excuse for a nurse who is dealing with a patient's eye injuries failing to notice that the size or reflex of his pupils is changing or that his conscious level is deteriorating, both of which are important pointers to rising intracranial pressure. An ophthalmic nurse who fails to notice that her patient is becoming pale, sweaty and drowsy or incoherent and to suspect clinical shock is failing in her duty to that patient. Any changes in the patient's condition, no matter how apparently trivial, should be recorded and reported at once so that any necessary treatment may commence. Any dramatic deterioration may call for the carrying out of emergency 'first aid' measures until help arrives; for example, the patient who suddenly loses consciousness should be turned onto his side and any dentures removed, and suction apparatus should be made readily available. The ophthalmic nurse who is aware of and prepared for the complications which may arise in injured patients is more likely to note the signs in good time and avoid endangering her patient's life.

FURTHER READING

Miller, S.J.H. (1984) *Parsons' Diseases of the Eye*, 17th Edn. Edinburgh: Churchill Livingstone.

16 Removal of the eye

'Pop', as he liked to be called, was confused and irritable when he was admitted to the ward. He had been a patient many times before as he suffered with glaucoma, but he had always been alert and gentle. He had just returned from a holiday with his daughter, which they had cut short because he had become so difficult and argumentative.

Pop said his eye was extremely painful and several retrobulbar injections of alcohol did little to relieve the pain. His intra-ocular pressure was very high and since no useful vision remained, it was decided that it should be removed.

Pop was helped to sit up in bed before his daughter visited the day after surgery. His first words to her were 'Janet, I can't tell you how wonderful it is—there's no more pain'. His confusion and irritability seemed to disappear with his eye!

Tom Smith had been assaulted and had needed many stitches in his face. His right eye had been lacerated and the cornea and sclera perforated. Surgical repair had been undertaken, but two days later it was clear that the repair was unsuccessful and the eye would have to be removed.

Tom had been very quiet and withdrawn since his admission and when the surgeon mentioned removing the eye he began to weep uncontrollably. It was several hours before he was able to discuss his feelings of horror, disgust and fear at the prospect of losing his eye. He was convinced that his wife would leave him and his friends would mock. He had been proud of his good looks and felt they would be ruined—he really wondered if life would be tolerable again.

ENUCLEATION

Enucleation of the eye involves removal of the whole eye with a small portion of the optic nerve but leaving the conjunctiva, bulbar fascia and the extrinsic muscles. It is indicated for:

(1) a painful blind eye;
(2) malignancies of the globe;
(3) severe injury to the eye where restoration of adequate function is impossible;
(4) preventing the development of sympathetic ophthalmitis.

EVISCERATION

This procedure involves removal of the contents of the eye but retaining the posterior part of the sclera so that the optic nerve remains intact, thus minimizing the risk of infection spreading to the brain. This method is sometimes used for the removal of a badly infected eye, but advances in antibiotic therapy have reduced the need for such measures.

EXENTERATION

Exenteration is a mutilating procedure which entails removal of the entire orbital contents including lids, eye and the orbital section of the optic nerve. It is used to prevent the spread of malignant tumours of the lacrimal gland, eyelids, conjunctiva and extensive intra-orbital tumours.

The exposed bony orbit is usually covered with a split skin graft and a prosthesis representing eyelids and an eye is fitted onto a spectacle frame.

NURSING CONSIDERATIONS

PRE-OPERATIVE CARE

The physical preparation for surgery to remove an eye is as for any other surgery with any local treatment continuing up to the time of operation. The affected eye should be clearly marked to avoid any chance of error.

Some patients will experience intense pain in their affected eye and effective pain control is a priority in the pre-operative period. Prescribed analgesics should be given regularly. The nurse should not wait for the patient's pain to return before giving the next dose of drugs but rather ensure that they are given in time to prevent the return of pain. If this method is adopted, simple analgesics such as paracetamol may be sufficient. If pain is not controlled, the nurse should note and report this to the medical staff so that more effective alternatives may be prescribed. It should not be forgotten that the patient who is anxious and fearful is more likely to experience pain than the one who is relaxed and has come to terms with his condition. The skilled nurse may be able to reduce the need for analgesics in some patients by allowing them to express their worries and by ensuring that they fully understand the reasons for their pain and the necessity for their forthcoming operation. The amount of psychological care required will vary greatly with the patient's needs and perceptions. Pop and Tom (see profiles above) represent two vastly differing attitudes—one only too pleased to be rid of his painful blind eye, the other regarding it as the end of meaningful life. The nurse should ensure that she makes time available to her patients and follows up any attempt they may make to discuss their worries and apprehensions.

When such mutilative surgery is to be undertaken, it is essential that the patient gives his *informed* consent to operation. While it is the doctor's duty to gain this consent, it is the nurse who is likely to be approached by the patient, who has not fully understood what is to happen or who feels uncertain as to whether he will or should have consented. The nurse should answer his questions and discuss the operation to the best of her ability, but should also ensure that the patient speaks again to the medical staff so that everyone is satisfied that fully informed consent has been given.

Once the need for removal is accepted, the patient may wish to express his fears about prostheses and his ability to handle them—for some the idea is utterly repugnant. It may be helpful if a visit from an ex-patient who is coping well following similar surgery can be arranged, or if the patient can handle an artificial eye.

Wherever possible, the patient's spouse, or parents in the case of children, or any other relative whom the patient should wish, should be involved in the pre-operative discussions about surgery and prostheses. Tom (see profile) was worried about how his wife would accept him with only one eye. Relatives will have worries about the surgery and the future implications, and will come to terms with their loved one's disfigurement more readily if given the opportunity to discuss it with the patient, nursing and medical staff prior to surgery. Their acceptance and support can be of great help to the patient at what may be an extremely difficult time.

POST-OPERATIVE CARE

A firm dressing will be applied to the socket in theatre to avoid haematoma formation. In addition to the general care required by any patient post-operatively, the nurse should observe the dressing for staining and report this if it occurs. Extra padding should be applied if necessary and the dressing left untouched for 24–48 hours.

Once the dressing is removed for the first time, the socket should be cleaned and redressed two or three times daily until any discharge has ceased when it may be left uncovered. The patient will be very conscious of his appearance at this stage, and may wish to wear dark glasses or to have the lens of his own spectacles covered.

Patients who have lost part of their body often go through a grieving process similar to that following bereavement. The nurse should be aware that this is likely, and able to reassure the patient that his feelings of anger or of not wanting to talk to anyone are quite natural at such a time. Each patient will accept the facts and come to terms with them in his own way and his own time, and no attempt should be made to force him to 'snap out of it'.

PROSTHESES

During surgery a plastic implant may be inserted into the socket and the four recti muscles sutured to it. This will allow some movement of the artificial eye. Others will return from theatre with a temporary shell in the socket, while yet others have nothing.

All patients will be prescribed an artificial eye, shaped and painted to their own requirements. Patients should be encouraged to handle both shells and artificial eyes (Fig. 16.1) so that they become familiar with them. They will also need reassurance that insertion, wearing and removal of these prostheses is not painful.

The patient should be seated for insertion of the prosthesis, which is moistened to facilitate its movement into the socket. The upper lid is raised and the upper edge of the prosthesis slipped under it and held in place with a thumb while the lower lid is drawn down and the lower edge of the prosthesis slipped into the lower fornix (Fig. 16.2).

Removal is achieved by asking the seated patient to look up and slipping a glass rod or finger under the lower edge of the prosthesis with the lower lid drawn down. Gentle pressure on the upper lid will then push the eye out.

The patient will need to be competent at these tasks before discharge, and the nurse will need patience, care and understanding when teaching him. At first, practice should be undertaken

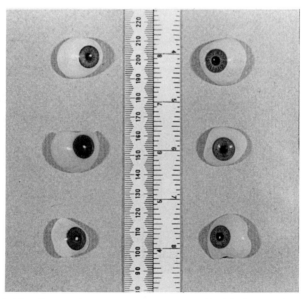

Fig. 16.1 *Prosthetic eyes, in various shapes and sizes according to the individual socket.*

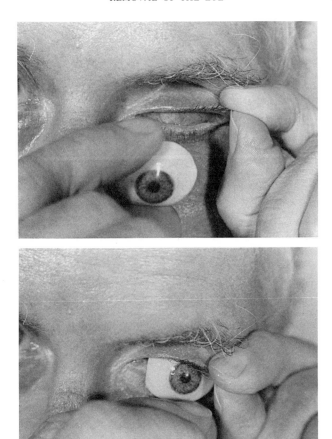

Fig. 16.2 *Inserting an artificial eye. (a) The upper eyelid is raised. (b) The artificial eye is inserted under the upper eyelid. The lower eyelid is then drawn down slightly and the prosthesis inserts into the socket.*

in privacy in front of a mirror with the surface in front of the patient covered with a towel in case he drops the eye. It may also be necessary or desirable to teach a relative to insert and remove the prosthesis. The nurse should be aware that it is often more difficult to perform such tasks on someone else, and should allow plenty of time and provide encouragement without trying to force participation before the relative is ready.

It is recommended that prostheses are removed at night and left in fresh water. In the morning, the socket should be gently cleaned and the eye reinserted.

FURTHER READING

Dorrell, E.D. (1978) *Surgery of the Eye*. Oxford. Blackwell Scientific.
Galbraith, J.E.K. (1979) *Basic Eye Surgery*. Edinburgh: Churchill Livingstone.
Lyle, T.K. & Cross, A.G. (1968) *May and Worth's Manual of Diseases of the Eye*. London: Baillière Tindall.
Miller, S.J.H. (1984) *Parsons' Diseases of the Eye*, 17th Edn. Edinburgh: Churchill Livingstone.

17 Out-patient and theatre nursing

OUT-PATIENT DEPARTMENT NURSING

Special skills are required of the ophthalmic nurse working in the out-patient department. Not least of these is the ability to establish a rapport with patients within a few minutes and an ability to inspire trust and confidence.

Because ophthalmology is such a specialized field of medicine, many general practitioners (GPs) send their patients to the hospital for diagnosis and care. Likewise, many district nurses do not feel sufficiently confident to carry out eye treatments in the patient's home and the patients return each time a treatment is required, often daily or more in the acute stages. Many patients with ophthalmic conditions do not need to be admitted to hospital and their care is carried out from start to finish in the out-patient department. This means that large numbers of patients will be seen each day, some perhaps for only a few minutes, and the ophthalmic nurse must endeavour to make each one feel welcome and special.

Many of the patients will be elderly and may be confused by the large numbers of people around them. They may not immediately understand what is said to them, and may need help to find their way around the department, particularly if they need a variety of tests in different rooms. The nurse will need particular tact, understanding and patience in dealing with this group of patients, and must assure herself that they understand and can manage any treatment that needs to be carried out at home.

In many departments, instructions for any treatment necessary at home are printed on cards so that there is no chance of instructions being misunderstood. Ensure that either the patient himself can read the instructions or that there is someone at home who can read them for him. The nurse should read the instructions through to the patient and encourage him to ask about anything he does not understand.

In many ophthalmic out-patient departments, patients are required to undergo a number of ophthalmic tests. These are usually carried out in separate rooms so that the best use is made of equipment, and personnel. For some patients this will mean a very long stay in the department as they queue for the different tests. The nurse should try to make a mental note of such patients so that she can ensure that they know where to find the toilets, and so that they do not go without food and drink unnecessarily. A few words of explanation from time to time about the necessity for the tests, or the reason for any delay will make the patient realize that he has not been forgotten, and will often calm those who are becoming agitated at the amount of time they seem to be wasting.

Most departments will run specialized clinics such as glaucoma, contact lens, neurology or diabetic clinics. This system makes the best use of equipment and medical staff's time, and means that the nurse can become attuned to the care of the patients with a particular ophthalmic disorder. For the most part she will act in a supportive role, assisting the doctor and giving reassurance, explanations and instructions to the patient. She should also ensure that any queries the patient has are fully answered before he leaves the department. At the diabetic clinics, the nurse must be alert for signs of her patients becoming hypoglycaemic and be prepared to take the necessary corrective action. It is particularly important that these patients do not miss meals because of delays in the department.

The out-patient nurse will be expected to accompany patients and assist with specialized investigations in the department. In addition to those described in Chapter 3, fundus fluorescein angiography and laser therapy are worthy of mention.

FUNDUS FLUORESCEIN ANGIOGRAPHY

This technique is used to demonstrate abnormalities in the vascular structure of the fundus. Sodium fluorescein is injected intravenously, usually into the patient's arm, and its circulation through the retinal blood vessels is recorded with a fundus camera attached to a slit lamp. Areas of retinal ischaemia (reduced blood supply) where there is capillary blockage, will show as dark, underperfused areas on the angiogram. In those patients with diabetic retinopathy (see Chapter 18), the new weak blood vessels will leak the fluorescein dye through their walls. Normal retinal vessels are impermeable to the dye. In order to facilitate good fundus views, the patient's pupils will be widely dilated.

The nurse should be able to explain this test to her patient and answer his questions. No anaesthetic is necessary and the procedure is not painful, but many patients will be worried at the thought of having dye injected and at the large pieces of equipment used. They should also be warned that the dye will affect other tissues in their body and their skin will become yellowish for a day or two. The dye will also make urine test unreliable in diabetic patients as it will be excreted from the body by this route.

LASER TREATMENT

The first solar burn of the retina which resulted in a central scotoma was recorded in the seventeenth century, and from that time experimentation continued into the action of focusing sunlight onto eyes. Light coagulation was first used therapeutically in the 1940s and the high-pressure xenon lamp was used for photocoagulation in 1956.

In 1971 the argon laser (Light Amplification by Stimulated Emission of Radiation) became commercially available, and is used with excellent results in vascular disease of the retina. In diabetic retinopathy, leaking vessels can be sealed or extensive areas of the peripheral retina treated. This alters the metabolic requirements of the retina in a manner which causes regression of new blood vessels found in proliferative retinopathy (see Chapter 18). Exudates at the macular area can be resolved or partly resolved using laser treatment.

More recently, the YAG (Yttrium–Aluminium–Garnet) laser, which creates lightning, has become available. This has opened up a whole new dimension in ophthalmic therapy, as the laser energy can be used to cut through transparent tissues such as the anterior and posterior lens capsule or membranes of the vitreous. This means that patients who previously would have required surgery can now be treated in the out-patient department.

Patients presenting for laser treatment for the first time will be naturally fearful of exactly what will happen to them. The ophthalmic nurse should be ready to explain in simple terms what will be done, and to assure her patient that the process is painless. The pupil will be dilated so that good retinal views may be obtained, and some patients will have the eye anaesthetized so that a contact lens can be placed on the eye to allow a wide angle view of the retina. Retrobulbar anaesthetic is sometimes necessary in a small number of patients who are unable to keep their eye still.

The out-patient ophthalmic nurse should ensure that she fulfils her role of maintaining links between her department and the community health workers, particularly the GPs and district nursing staff. Home visits may be needed once the patient has been discharged from the care of the hospital staff, and good communications will ensure that the staff in the community know precisely what treatment the patient has received and how his care should continue.

The ophthalmic nurse in the out-patient department must ensure that her clinical knowledge is up to date and that her nursing skills are competent. She will require a certain amount of technical knowledge in order to help maintain and use the many pieces of equipment she will find in the department. In addition, she will need to develop her skills of management if she is to be an effective team member in a well-run department, and her public relations skills if she is to make each of her many patients feel that she cares about them.

OPHTHALMIC THEATRE NURSING

Ophthalmic theatre nursing is a very specialized part of ophthalmic nursing. The intricate and delicate work done on the eye requires particularly high standards of care on the part of all the theatre staff. Infection transferred to the eye may lead to blindness or loss of that eye, and standards of cleanliness must be strict and scrupulous. Many of the instruments used in ophthalmic surgery are very delicate and must be carefully looked after and maintained. A nurse who is clumsy in laying out her instruments may easily damage them.

As far as possible, nursing care in theatre must be continuous with that which the patient receives on the ward both prior to and following his operation. In many hospitals, a nurse from the ward will accompany the patient into the theatre anaesthetic room and stay with him until he is fully anaesthetized. In other hospitals, the patient will be received in a transfer area by a theatre nurse who will care for him until anaesthesia is induced. If this is the policy of the hospital, the theatre nurse should try to visit the patient on the previous day so that her face is familiar. She may spend a few minutes introducing herself and telling the patient what to expect in theatre.

The nurse should remain with her patient until he is anaesthetized. She should reassure her patient if he expresses any fears but should allow him to relax under the influence of his premedication drugs if possible. The patient should be made as comfortable as possible on the theatre trolley. The nurse may wish to make a final check that all necessary pre-operative nursing tasks have been completed, including removal of any prostheses from the patient, taping of rings and completion of any paperwork.

If the operation is to be performed under local anaesthetic, the nurse will stay with her patient throughout. Some patients find it helpful to hold the nurse's hand, particularly if she is outside their visual field, others find it helpful to chat to the nurse in order to direct their thoughts from the operative procedure. Never assume that a patient wants to talk or be touched, but let him know that you are there to help in whatever way he wishes.

If the patient has received a general anaesthetic, the theatre nurse should ensure that he is positioned correctly on the operating table with all his limbs in a natural position. The position of the patient's head will be of particular importance in the ophthalmic theatre. She should also ensure that no part of the patient is touching the metal parts of the table since pressure sores can readily occur during a long operation and there is a risk of the patient receiving burns if diathermy is used during surgery.

In the recovery period, the patient should be placed in a suitable position, usually on his side with the operated eye uppermost. Following surgery for retinal detachment, the surgeon may request that the patient be nursed in a particular position in order to aid healing of the retina; this may mean that extra precautions are necessary to maintain patency of the patient's airway. The

patient's respiratory rate, pulse, blood pressure and skin colour
should be observed and recorded regularly until he is fully conscious and the observations are all within normal limits. The
surgeon should be notified at once of any deterioration in his
patient's condition. Analgesics should be given as prescribed to
relieve any pain or discomfort that the patient may feel. Vomiting
should be avoided as this can cause damage to the operated eye,
and anti-emetics should be given if the patient feels nauseated or
if opiate drugs are given, since these are known to cause vomiting
in some individuals. Suction apparatus should be readily available
at the patient's bedside so that any excessive secretions in the
nose or mouth may be removed quickly.

The nurse should talk to her patient as he recovers, reminding
him where he is and what has happened and encouraging him to
remain in any required position. She should ensure that he is
comfortable, warm and pain-free.

The theatre nurse will hand the patient back to the care of the
ward staff and should ensure that nursing records are up to date
and that any informtion relevant to the future care of the patient
is clearly understood.

FURTHER READING

Brigden, R.J. (1980) *Operating Theatre Technique*. Edinburgh: Churchill Living-
stone.
Dixon, E. (1983) *Theatre Technique*. London: Baillière Tindall.
L'Esperance, F.A. Jr (1983) *Ophthalmic Lasers*. 2nd Edn. London: C.V. Mosby.

18 The eye and general health

George Watson was a 54-year-old joiner who was presented in the casualty department because one morning he was unable to see clearly. His visual acuity was greatly reduced in both eyes. His vision had been blurred in one eye for about three weeks but he had not been worried until the second eye became affected.

When questioned about his general health, he admitted to getting breathless sometimes and to increasingly frequent headaches. Mr Watson's blood pressure was found to be 240/120 mmHg, and when his pupils were dilated and his fundi examined using an ophthalmoscope severe hypertensive retinopathy was apparent. The findings were explained to Mr Watson and he was transferred at once to a medical ward for treatment of his hypertension.

DEVELOPMENT OF THE EYE

The embryological development of the eye begins early and may be noted at about three weeks' gestation when the site of the eye is indicated by a flattened area on both sides of the anterior end of the neural groove. The flattened area gradually becomes cupped and the retina and lens begin to form by about four weeks. At three months the secondary lens fibres can be seen and eyelid folds develop. By four months, the sphincter and dilator muscles of the iris are forming, as are the sclera and choroid, the ciliary muscle and the central retinal artery. The eye looks almost normal at this stage, although medullation of the optic nerve fibres does not begin until about seven months' gestation and is completed only shortly before birth.

The eye does not function in isolation but as an important sensory organ of the body. It depends on the body for its nutrition carried to it by circulating blood and, in return, it supplies the body with vital information about its surroundings. In its complex structure, the eye contains cells representative of most body tissues—epithelial, muscles, blood, connective tissue and nerve cells—and many diseases which affect other tissues of the body also affect the eye.

CARDIOVASCULAR DISEASE AND THE EYE

HYPERTENSION

A number of ophthalmic changes will occur in the patient with uncontrolled hypertension, such as irregular narrowing of those vessels, and this is often accompanied by haemorrhages in the nerve fibre layers, retinal oedema, and the formation of fluffy white patches ('cotton wool patches') in the nerve fibre layer of the retina. Papilloedema and occlusion of the large retinal arteries occur in severe cases, and are often irreversible.

ATHEROMA

Atheromatous changes may lead to carotid artery ischaemia and the shooting off of small emboli (due to irregular lining of the vessel walls) into the ophthalmic artery. This causes *amaurosis fugax*, transient loss of vision in one eye. The pupillary light reflex is absent but returns, with vision, after a few minutes. Treatment is with low doses of aspirin which acts as an anticoagulant, and the patient may require surgery to remove the atheromatous plaques from the carotid artery.

BLOOD DISORDERS

Anaemias leave the retina short of red blood cells and it appears pale when viewed through an ophthalmoscope. In severe anaemias haemorrhages may occur in the retina and choroid. The conjunctivae often appear pale and are commonly used as an indicator when anaemia is suspected.

The hyperviscosity associated with *polycythaemia* (an excess of red blood cells) results in retinal veins which are dark, tortuous and dilated and may haemorrhage. Conjunctival blood vessels will also be dilated. Similar changes may be noted in sufferers of *sickle cell anaemia*, in which sickled erythrocytes block capillaries and cause blood stasis and anoxia to small areas of the eye.

CONNECTIVE TISSUE DISEASE AND THE EYE

Also known as collagen diseases, this group of disorders is characterized by widespread inflammatory damage to connective tissue with fibrin deposits. It is probable that the body produces antibodies to its own tissues.

Lupus erythematosus, a chronic skin disease, may produce patchy erythema and atrophy of the skin of the eyelids. The most common ocular complication is severe retinopathy, with cotton wool patches and widespread retinal haemorrhages.

Rheumatoid arthritis is a chronic inflammatory disease of the joints. It is a disease of middle and old age, more common in women. Scleritis may occur in sufferers and the sclera may become thin and rupture and destroy the eye. Many patients with rheumatoid arthritis have dry eye syndrome (see Chapter 8). An added problem is the difficulty the patient has in holding the drop bottles to instil the artificial tears.

Marfan's syndrome is a genetic abnormality of connective tissue, resulting in aortic dilatation commonly preceding dissecting aneurysm, and multiple skeletal defects, notably excessive length of the long bones. Eye manifestations include subluxation of the lens, which may be small and have a cataract. The anterior chamber angle may be deformed and patients tend to be myopic and have bright blue sclera. They are also prone to develop retinal detachment.

ENDOCRINE DISORDERS AND THE EYE

HYPERTHYROIDISM (GRAVES'S DISEASE)

An excessive production of thyroid hormones causes widespread neuromuscular changes and increased tissue metabolism. Systemic manifestations include fatigue, weight loss despite an increased food intake, tachycardia, and heat intolerance accompanied by excessive sweating. More than 50% of patients with hyperthyroid-ism develop eye signs.

Exophthalmos is the most striking eye change; the eyes become abnormally prominent. Exophthalmos is usually bilateral in thy-roid disease, though often more marked on one side. The eyes become sensitive to light, with irritable conjunctiva. The eyelids may not entirely cover the globe and keratitis resulting in visual loss may result if the cornea is not protected.

Orbital congestion is common. The puffy eyelids and chemosed, injected conjunctiva are readily visible, and epiphora may result from marked conjunctival oedema. Severe orbit congestion may limit eye movement and this may be compounded by contracture of the extra-ocular muscles. There may also be optic nerve com-pression. These complications are treated with large doses of systemic steroids, and with orbital decompression or radiation therapy if the steroid therapy fails.

DIABETES MELLITUS

This metabolic disorder results from abnormal insulin production, and may occur in individuals of any age. It has a number of ocular manifestations, notably a typical retinopathy. Senile cataract is likely to develop 10 years earlier in the elderly diabetic person than in the non-diabetic population.

The factors affecting diabetic retinopathy are multiple. The severity of diabetic retinopathy depends on the duration of the disease and the adequacy of its control, particularly in the first five years of the disease. It does not depend on the severity of the diabetes. Pathological changes occur in the retinal vessels, and the inner part of the retina is most affected. Multiple retinal microaneurysms occur and are followed by small dark haemor-rhages. In more advanced cases new vessels begin to bud from the veins (neovascularization) and grow over the retinal surface and disc. They can bleed into the vitreous, thus causing vitreous haemorrhage and retinal detchment and so blindness. Visual acu-ity is a poor indicator of the severity of this type of retinopathy; if the fovea centralis is unaffected there may be excellent vision despite advanced retinal changes, whereas a single lesion involving the fovea may markedly reduce vision.

Diabetes is thought to have a heredity causal factor, though this is unproven. Some GPs regularly screen those patients with a family history of diabetes so that any signs of the disease appearing are detected at an early stage. Diabetic physicians will examine the eyes of all their patients regularly in order that diabetic retinopathy can be identified at an early stage.

SKIN DISORDERS AND THE EYE

ALBINISM

Albinism is an inherited disorder of the pigment cell system in the skin. Low levels or absence of melanin results in a fair complexion, blonde hair and poor vision. The fundus may appear blonde, although patchy pigmented areas at the periphery are common. Because the retinal pigment epithelium cannot absorb light, the fovea centralis fails to develop and visual acuity is reduced. In infants, the iris is pale grey and translucent so that red light is reflected from the fundus. Nystagmus and squint are common, but the outstanding symptom is photophobia and sufferers are extremely intolerant of light. Good vision is usually possible with the aid of tinted corrective spectacles.

ACNE ROSACEA

This common skin disease is frequently associated with conjunctivitis and sometimes keratitis. The typical flushing of the skin of the cheeks may extend to the lids, causing scaly desquamation and hyperaemia.

HERPES ZOSTER OPHTHALMICUS

This extremely painful condition is most common in people over the age of 50 who have had chicken pox in the past. Some of the virus remains in the trigeminal nerve ganglia and may reactivate years later to produce the typical lesions of *Herpes zoster* (see Fig. 18.1).

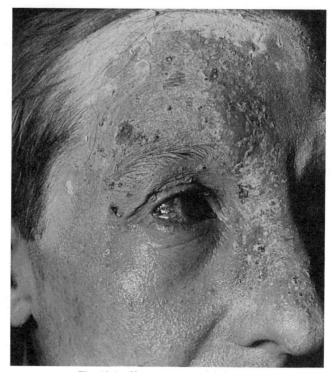

Fig. 18.1 *Herpes zoster ophthalmicus.*

A flu-like illness precedes severe pain along the distribution of the ophthalmic nerve—the scalp, forehead, upper eyelid and tip of the nose. The skin becomes red and a rash develops; vesicles turn to pustules and eventually crusts form after about 10 days. The conjunctiva usually becomes red and keratitis may occur. Iritis and secondary glaucoma may also occur.

Following *Herpes zoster* the cornea may remain anaesthetic and the consequences must be explained to the patient.

The main problem for most patients with *Herpes zoster* is the intense pain which accompanies it, particularly in the early stages. Effective pain control is vital if complications such as severe depression, loss of appetite and inability to sleep are to be avoided. Assessment of each patient's pain level and the effect of prescribed analgesics must be undertaken, since there is such a variety of experience with this condition. Some individuals may require pethidine or dihydrocodeine to control pain in the early stages while others find paracetamol effective. Analgesics should be taken regularly and before further pain is experienced; four-hourly doses will usually suffice. Night sedation may be necessary in the early stages, and patients who suffer loss of appetite should be offered nourishing drinks during this period. The patient should be helped to feel as much in control of his condition as possible. This may be achieved by allowing him to control his own analgesia, ensuring that he knows how and where to seek help when he feels particularly low, but above all by ensuring that he understands and is prepared to cope with the likely symptoms and effects of this condition. A small number of patients suffer intense neuralgic pain for years, become very depressed and may even attempt suicide. Antidepressants may be required, and the nurse will need to offer her patients constant reassurance that the condition will ultimately improve.

The skin lesions are generally treated with an antiviral paint such as Herpid paint for five days, and then with an antibiotic ointment to decrease the risk of infection. Where the cornea is involved, acyclovir ointment or a similar antiviral agent will be indicated, as will the use of antibiotic and mydriatic eye drops. Tarsorrhaphy will be carried out once the skin lesions have healed if the cornea becomes insensitive.

NEUROLOGICAL DISORDERS AND THE EYE

MULTIPLE SCLEROSIS

This chronic disease is characterized by disseminated areas of demyelination of nerve sheaths. Eye symptoms include retrobulbar neuritis and paresis of one or more ocular muscles, leading to diplopia. Nystagmus is common in the later stages of the disease.

INTRACRANIAL LESIONS

Tumours, abscesses, aneurysms and haemorrhages within the brain may all interfere with nerve transmission to and from the eyes. The area of reduced vision will depend on the site of the lesion; for example, bitemporal hemianopia (loss of the temporal field of vision in both eyes) will result from a pituitary tumour which impinges on the optic chiasma. Papilloedema will occur as a result of raised intracranial pressure, and extra-ocular muscles paresis may occur.

VITAMIN DEFICIENCIES AND THE EYE

VITAMIN A

Deficiency of vitamin A will cause softening and drying of the cornea (keratomalacia). This can lead to blindness if infection results and the cornea disintegrates. Night blindness is one of the first symptoms of the disease but, since vitamin deficiencies occur more commonly in children, may not be noticed. The condition is still common in many parts of Africa and Asia and usually accompanies generalized malnutrition. Urgent treatment with massive doses of vitamin A is essential if rapidly developing blindness is to be avoided.

VITAMIN B

Deficiency of vitamin B may give rise to bilateral optic neuritis and defective day vision, particularly in those patients who derive most of their calories from alcohol. Visual acuity may be reduced to 6/60, but will improve if vitamin B is provided.

DRUG ABUSE AND THE EYE

Endogenous *Candida* endophthalmitis represents one of the most serious ocular complications of intravenous drug abuse. *Candida* is a yeast-like fungus which is probably spread intravenously in the drug abuser following injection with unsterile needles. It is not clear why the eye should be specially liable to infection.

The fungus enters the eye from a chorioretinal focus and spreads to the vitreous where it proliferates. The foci appear as small

white fluffy areas on the retinal surface, and typical acc
in the vitreous ('string of pearls') may also be seen. Unt
red eye is present at the beginning and this proceeds to p.
photophobia, scleritis, retinochoroiditis and finally to inflammatory response within the vitreous, leading to visual loss.

The patients tend not to present in the ophthalmic department
until they are in severe pain or are frightened by the loss of vision;
by this time the condition is well established and the patient will
need hospitalization for treatment. This can cause many nursing
problems, as patients may be hepatitis and/or AIDS carriers,
aggressive and abusive, uncooperative and devious, particularly
where drugs are concerned. Policies on withdrawal or continuation
of drugs will vary from hospital to hospital, and both medical and
nursing staff will need to work closely with the team from the
local drug dependency clinic.

Antifungal drugs will be administered by intra-vitreal injection
and by intravenous infusion. Systemic steroids may also be
required.

Many of these patients refuse to stay in hospital for the desired
time, and treatment stops when they discharge themselves. There
is little, if any, follow-up since they generally fail to attend out-
patient clinics.

FURTHER READING

Miller, S.J.H. (1984) *Parsons' Diseases of the Eye*, 17th Edn. Edinburgh: Churchill
Livingstone.
Servant, J.B., Dutton, G.N., Ong-Tone, L., Barrie, T. & Davey, C. (1985)
Candidal endophthalmitis in Glaswegian heroin addicts: report of an epi-
demic. *Transactions of the Ophthalmological Societies of The United King-
dom*, **104** (3), 297–308.

ree-quarters of the 100 000 registered blind
f 70 years, with the commonest causes being
catara~   a and senile degeneration of the macula. The
statutory definition of blindness is that 'a person should be so
blind as to be unable to perform any work for which eyesight is
essential'. Only about 10% of those registered as blind are unable
to see anything at all, or to differentiate between light and dark.

A person may be registered as partially sighted, and be entitled
to use the services appropriate to blind people, or partially sighted
and unlikely to deteriorate. There is no statutory definition of
partial sight.

The Certificate of Registration of Blindness (form BD8 in
England & Wales and BP1 in Scotland) is completed by the
consultant ophthalmologist after he has examined the patient.
Registration is voluntary, the completed form being sent to the
Director of Social Services for the area in which the patient lives.
The local authority will inform the patient of the facilities available
to them. Many of these services are organized through the Royal
National Institute for the Blind (RNIB).

SERVICES FOR YOUNG BLIND PEOPLE

Every year the sight of a number of children deteriorates through
the progression of a sight defect, or through illness or accident.
Those who are born blind or whose sight deteriorates at an early
age will stay at home to be cared for by their families. Advisers
from the RNIB or the local authority will provide practical help
and support to these families so that the child becomes an inte-
grated member of the community. Blind children need extra care
if they are to develop normally. They will need to develop the
senses of smell, hearing and touch to help to compensate for
their lack of sight, and will need particular encouragement with
speaking since they are unable to associate words with viewed
objects around them.

The family members will require a great deal of support to adapt to their child's disability. They will want to know what sort of local provisions and help are available for them and their child, and the ophthalmic nurse should ensure that she is able to put them in touch with appropriate agencies. Families should be given accurate and realistic guidance as to what help they can expect both immediately and in the future.

Some children will be able to attend ordinary schools if given adequate support, but others will do better by being with other visually handicapped children in a specialist school. The Sunshine House Nursery Schools are residential and take children from the age of about three and a half until they are ready for primary education.

There are specialist schools for the blind at both primary and secondary level, but most have links with local sighted schools and encourage pupils to transfer to them if at all possible. A number of specialist schools are run for those with other handicaps in addition to their blindness, and some hospitals have special residential units for such children.

School leavers who are not undertaking higher education may need specialist careers advice or further training. A number of educational and training courses are run by the RNIB, and many local authorities are setting up small units within their colleges of further education to cater for the visually handicapped and to increase the student's independence and confidence. RNIB advisers will help with preparations for employment and with finding a suitable job at the end of the course.

SERVICES FOR ADULT BLIND PEOPLE

Newly blind adults will need special care and support as they orientate themselves and adjust to their disability and the changes in lifestyle that it entails. Local authority social services departments will help with mastering new techniques for dealing with day-to-day activities and getting about without sight. The two main aids to mobility are the long white cane or stick with which blind people are issued, and guide dogs, which are available to a minority of blind patients through the Guide Dogs for the Blind Association, 113 Uxbridge Road, London W5. Wherever possible, newly blind persons are encouraged to attend a residential centre where, in addition, they can learn to read and write braille or Moon and to touch type.

Many blind people are employed on equal terms in offices and industry with sighted people. Help is available through the Manpower Services Commission to provide assessment for future training and employment and to provide 'on-the-job' training to ensure that the blind employee can do his work safely and efficiently.

Other blind adults need sheltered employment which is provided in special workshops and in homeworkers schemes administered by local authorities or voluntary societies for the blind. Most of these carry out light engineering and assembly processes, and very few continue the traditional crafts of basket and brush making.

Piano tuning has become a well established occupation for blind people, and can be lucrative as well as providing scope for those wishing to be self-employed. The RNIB provides courses for this and for those wishing to enter commercial or professional work. A range of special equipment is available to help blind people at work and can be provided through the Employment Services Commission.

St Dunstan's offers help to blind people who have served in the armed forces, and to firemen, policemen and nurses blinded on duty.

Residential homes are available for blind persons, but the number of places is limited. Demand for more accommodation is increasing with the rise in the number of elderly blind people, and homes to provide care are being adapted or purpose-built.

Many people who become blind are concerned about their financial position. A wide range of benefits is available from the Department of Health and Social Security, e.g. disablement benefit and mobility allowance. If these are insufficient for the needs of the blind person and his family, he may claim supplementary benefit which is payable at a higher rate to those registered blind. Extra income tax relief is allowed and additional financial assistance may be available through voluntary agencies.

Travel concessions are available in some areas, and guide dogs are sometimes allowed to travel free.

Reading materials including newspapers, periodicals and books for purchase or loan are available in both braille and Moon. A braille edition of the *Radio Times* is available free. For those with poor sight, large print books are available from most public libraries.

Talking books, recorded by professional readers, are light-weight cassettes which may be played on special playback machines. They are available through the RNIB's Talking Book Library and the annual subscription is usually paid by the local authority. A number of talking newspapers are also available. Portable radios are available through the British Wireless for the Blind Fund and a television sound-only receiver is available, for which a licence is not needed.

Many games and appliances have been devised for the blind. These include braille playing cards, watches and clocks with raised markings, and needle threaders. Braille dials and buttons are available for almost all cookers and washing machines (Fig. 19.1).

Holiday homes and accommodation for the blind are available through the RNIB and some local authorities and voluntary organizations.

Since services and provisions vary so widely from one area to another, the ophthalmic nurse should find out exactly what is available in her local area. She should develop as many contacts as possible with the helping agencies and personnel so that she is able realistically to advise her patients and tell them how to make contact.

NURSING CONSIDERATIONS

Nursing blind patients in a hospital ward or clinic presents special challenges and rewards for the nurse.

On admission to the ward, the blind patient may be very confused by the unfamiliar surroundings, and the nurse should ensure that he is adequately orientated to his new environment. He should be guided around the relevant areas as many times as necessary, and the positions of furniture and doors carefully explained. He will probably wish to feel these articles in order improve his mental image of the ward. When guiding a blind person, always allow them to take your arm and lead them, do not push them from behind. Always give clear instructions about

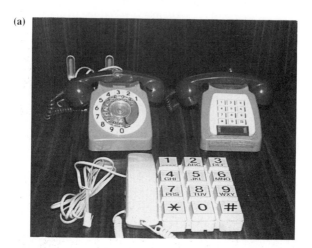

(a)

(b)

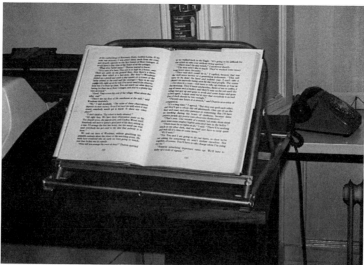

Fig. 19.1 *(a) Available telephones: machines with dials have clear letters on a white background, while the press-button telephone has very large raised numbers compared with the normal press-button telephone. (b) Stand for large print books. (c) Magnifying glass on stand to aid with reading. (d) Low visual aids – magnifying glasses.*

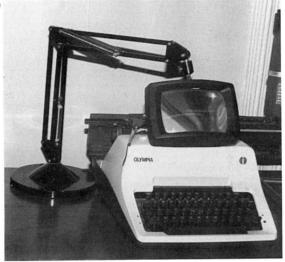

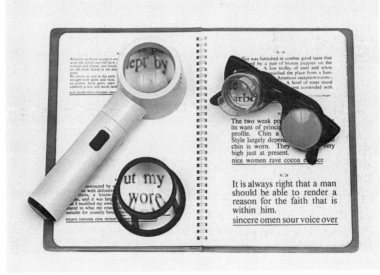

any obstacles or potential hazards such as low lights or steps.

When talking to a blind person, remember to tell them your name and status, and make it plain when you are terminating the conversation and leaving them. It can be humiliating to find yourself taking to thin air and it happens very easily to blind patients.

Each patient will have different needs and they will vary in their confidence and ability to get about. The nurse should assess the potential of each individual and ensure that he achieves that potential as far as possible within the given situation. The best person to ask about how much they can see and what help they need is the patient himself. Never force a patient to accept help, unless he is clearly a danger to himself or others. As a general rule, patients who are newly blind will need more help from the nursing staff than those who have already learned to cope with their disability.

A partially sighted patient will feel much more comfortable in the ward if he is provided with aids appropriate to his visual requirements. Some of these may be brought in from his home; others will be available through the hospital services.

Meals can present a problem for some blind patients if the nurse is thoughtless in her presentation. The meal should be placed in front of the patient, who may wish to place his hand on the rim of the plate. The nurse should explain what is being served and the relative position of each item on the plate; for example, 'meat is at 3 o'clock, potatoes are at 12 o'clock, carrots at 9 o'clock'. The patient may prefer his food to be cut up for him or may prefer to eat with a spoon—never assume this or you may cause offence. If a blind patient needs to be fed, indicate what is in each mouthful, and tell him when he is eating the last mouthful of one course or the first mouthful of the next.

When dispensing medication to blind or partially sighted patients, the nurse should place the tablets or medicine pot in the patient's hand and tell him what he is taking and how many tablets there are. Clear instructions must be given when the patient is discharged with medication to be taken at home, and the use of individual dose tablet dispensers may be appropriate for some patients—some of these are available with days and times printed in braille.

Guide dogs and their owners need to maintain contact, and

hospital admission can be distressing for both. Facilities should be made available for the dogs to visit if at all possible, but nursing staff should resist the temptation to pet and play with them since they are working dogs.

Some blind patients will have other disabilities in addition and will need extra care. Many blind patients are elderly and may be deaf in addition, and communication with them can present problems. The nurse should familiarize herself with the methods of writing letters on the palm of a deaf-and-blind person's hand, or with the manual alphabet.

Many useful leaflets relating to services and methods of assisting blind people are available through the following organizations:

Royal National Institute for the Blind,
224 Great Portland Street, London, W1N 6AA
Tel: 01–388 1266

The Partially Sighted Society,
40 Wordsworth Street, Hove, East Sussex, BN3 5BH
Tel: (0273) 736053

The Southern and Western Regional Association for the Blind,
55 Eton Avenue, London, NW3 3ET
Tel: 01–586 5655

The North Regional Association for the Blind,
Headingley Castle, Headingley Lane, Leeds, LS6
Tel: (0532) 752666

The Optical Information Council,
Walter House, 418–422 The Strand, London, WC2R OPB
Tel.: 01–836 2323

RCN Association of Nursing Practice,
Royal College of Nursing of the United Kingdom,
20 Cavendish Square, London, W1M OAB
Tel: 01–409 3333

Resource Centre for the Blind,
276 St Vincent Street, Glasgow, G2 5RP
Tel: 041–248 5811

FURTHER READING

Klemz, A. (1977) *Blindness and Partial Sight*. Cambridge: Woodhead-Faulkner.

20 Individualized nursing care

by Brigid Knight

'The unique function of the nurse is to assist the individual, sick or well, in the performance of those activities contributing to health or its recovery (or to a peaceful death) that he would perform unaided if he had the necessary strength, will or knowledge, and to do this in such a way as to help him to gain independence as rapidly as possible.'

Virginia Henderson (1966)

The acquisition of knowledge is useless unless it is applied effectively to the care of patients. A speciality such as ophthalmic nursing requires not only a good knowledge base but efficient planning and delivery of care: inconsistency only increases anxiety levels in patients and staff.

Since Virginia Henderson started to examine the concept of nursing, nurses have striven to perfect a way of identifying what nursing is, the framework around which care is planned, and the best way of identifying the care required by each individual.

The discussion about the nature of nursing continues, ever complicated by seemingly endless extension of the nurse's role, and will vary depending on the individual's own perception of their role.

The nursing process is almost universally accepted as the framework of care: its four stages, assessment, planning, implementation and evaluation, formally identify the facets of care that all nurses say they have carried out for years. This is probably true, although it might be suggested that traditional, ritualistic care did not always reflect the needs of the individual, but was based on a medical model, the care given being dependent on the diagnosis rather than the person.

The need for a process of care that could be documented and hence seen by all concerned has been enhanced by many things:

(1) A requirement to have a scientific, demonstrable basis that gives reasons for care, the intervention planned and its effectiveness.
(2) The degree to which nurses are now required to account for their own actions.
(3) The decrease in working hours, leading to less overlap between staff.
(4) An increase in staff turnover, related to the common problem of the trained : learner ratio.

In an area where the nursing process is used properly, it should be possible for a nurse to come on duty and have immediate access to enough documented information to give care effectively. This is especially important in areas such as ophthalmic units, where a high proportion of staff are not specialist trained and whose generalist knowledge may not be sufficient to give safe care. The process should be the basis for all nursing care, as it allows for the identification of problems, be they actual or potential, and for negotiation with the patient as to what they consider to be a priority. This has led to problems in past care plans that have been designed to alleviate the nurse's problems rather than the patient's, and so great has the discussion been that an alternative has now been proffered in the form of nursing diagnoses. There is also a danger that, in trying to anticipate problems, the nurse may place undue emphasis on certain aspects of care, causing the patient to expect the problem to develop—a self-fulfilling prophecy. Once the problems have been identified, possible solutions are implemented, but unfortunately this is often where the process stops.

The evaluation and updating of care are often neglected, leading to information that is out of date, so that either an unnecessary amount of care is given or, worse still, necessary care is omitted, because no reassessment of the situation has taken place.

In ophthalmic nursing this problem is compounded by the relatively short length of stay in hospital and the variation in degrees of dependence/independence, not only between individual patients but for the same person during their treatment.

Lack of time is often the reason given for bad evaluation techniques, but an initially well written care plan, regularly updated, will save time eventually because it reduces the need for constant reference to others for information, and the nurse giving the care will function more effectively knowing what is expected of her.

Having provided a systematic approach to planning and delivery of care, nursing models are the means of identifying the components of care, and they give a more definite understanding of the patient's needs and how they may be met. There are many models of nursing, some very similar, while others take a different perspective: it was Virginia Henderson who first tried to identify the fundamental needs that are common to all.

In 1970, Calista Roy instigated the use of a model that emphasized the individual's interaction with the environment. She felt that the nurse should only intervene when there was an inability on the part of the patient to adapt to the situation for whatever reason. It is then the nurse's role to manipulate the situation to remit or augment the elements that are causing the patient's inability to cope, or to help the patient overcome the cause of the deficit in adaptation.

In 1980, Dorothy Orem's self-care model was published: her philosophy was that an individual is responsible for his own health and well-being, and so the emphasis is on health rather than ill-health. It emphasizes the nurse's role as a health educator, and intervention is only required when the individual can no longer care for himself and there is a health care deficit, but only after family and significant others have been involved and yet the deficit still remains.

This is a very brief simplistic outline of two of the best known models, but on closer examination it becomes obvious that both require a degree of knowledge on the part of the nurse that perhaps learners or general nurses working in a specialist area such as ophthalmology do not possess. This may be because both models were developed in North America where nursing practice and economic demands result in different resources and needs. Both models are applicable to ophthalmic nursing: because of the emphasis on adaptation to a change in the individual's relationship with his environment, the Roy model may be useful in the rehabilitation of the visually handicapped; this also is true of the Orem model, because a philosophy of self-care encourages independence and the use of existing facilities.

Roper, Logan and Tierney (1980) developed a British model that has been said to be a modification of Henderson's original concept. They based their model on the premise that an illness is but an episode in life, and there should be minimal disturbance to the individual's activities of living while requiring nursing care. Many people do not look beyond the 12 activities of living that the model lists, but there are other elements described (Table 20.1). If they are all considered when using this model, many of the arguments against its use, such as the lack of psychological input, would be overcome. The advantage of this model seems to be that everyone experiences the activities of living, so that it only requires a basic knowledge to begin to formulate some idea of the problems, actual or potential, that may require nursing action.

When trying to decide which of the numerous models to use in any one clinical area, much will depend on the type of patient, the sort of goals to be achieved and the expertise of the staff. No model is sacrosanct, and there is much to be said for adapting basic ideas to suit the individual needs of the area.

Table 20.1 *Model From 'Elements of Nursing' by Roper, Logan & Tierney*

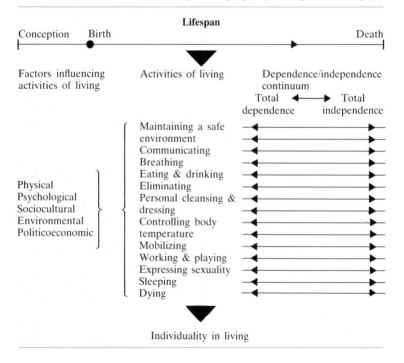

There are many arguments against the use of both the nursing process and nursing models; Gott (1988) noted that stress occurred when a nurse was unable to find a solution to a problem that she and the patient had identified. She felt that the careers needed support too if individualized patient care was to be carried out effectively. However, it is implicit in the process that some problems will be identified that are beyond the remit of the nurse, and there must be an awareness of this.

A greater stress may be caused if the problems are insoluble due to reasons that the nurse identifies as being avoidable, such as economic cutbacks and shortage of staff.

The question of the time it takes to assess a patient adequately and to write a care plan may be overcome by the use of standardized forms. These give the basic information applicable to certain types of patients, although the trap to be avoided is that of moving back to the medical model—the problems must be patient-orientated. The individual's special problems/needs are then added, and so hopefully a lot of repetitious writing is avoided. This could work well in an ophthalmic unit, as shown in Tables 20.2 and 20.3, care plans for specific ophthalmic pre- and post-operative care, based on, although not strictly adhering to, the Roper, Logan and Tierney model.

Another aspect of the use of the process and models in ophthalmic nursing is the implicit belief that care should be negotiated with the individual. Many elderly patients find this hard to accept; they come from a generation who saw doctors, and to some extent, nurses as infallible beings with total control and may find it difficult to become involved in discussions about their own care. The idea may need to be introduced gradually and, in some cases, the nurse should just draw up the plan and explain its significance, although it is important to make sure that the individual's reluctance to participate in his care is not due to lack of knowledge rather than anything else.

Conversely, the benefits of planning effective care on a logical, well thought out basis are infinite. The care of the ophthalmic patient, although a specialist subject, is potentially wide ranging, and using a model allows a picture of the needs of the whole person to be established.

The importance of individualized nursing care to the visually handicapped is paramount, and assists in the establishment of

Table 20.2 *Specific pre-operative care of patients undergoing intra-ocular surgery*

Patient's problems	Nursing intervention	Expected outcome
Anxiety Potential anxiety, due to: • Decreased vision or loss of independence	Explain that surgery should improve vision eventually; introduce them to patients who have had the same sort of operation	Relaxed patient, optimistic about the outcome of treatment
• New surroundings, and ignorance of what is expected of him	Orientate the patient and his family to the ward area and explain the routine	Well-orientated patient
• Fear of anaesthesia and surgery	Ensure they know exactly what is going to happen prior to, during and after surgery	Patient understands what is going to happen and what is expected of him
Maintaining a safe environment Potential wrong operation performed	Check that the correct eye has been marked by the surgeon, and that the consent has been signed	Patient has correct operation
Potential risk of infection	Eye lashes may be trimmed using curved scissors coated with Chloramphenicol ointment or petroleum jelly to prevent lash remnants dropping into the eye: instil prophylactic antimicrobial eyedrops as prescribed	Recovery not delayed by onset of infection

Potential injury from or damage to: dentures, contact lenses, hair clips, hearing aid, spectacles, prostheses	Remove everything except spectacles and hearing aids—these can be removed in the anaesthetic room: contact lenses *must* be removed before leaving the ward	Surgery/anaesthetic not complicated by inhalation of foreign body etc., but patient still able to communicate with all staff he meets prior to surgery
Potential risk of pre-operative complications	Instil drops prescribed by the surgeon prior to surgery, e.g. mydrilate, and give any appropriate prescribed systemic premedication	Operation is carried out safely
Elimination Anxiety about defaecation and passing urine post-operatively, and the effect of straining on the incisions	Check that the patient has had his bowels open within the previous 24 hours: offer a bedpan/bottle or ask patient if he wishes to go to the toilet just prior to premedication	Patient feels at ease and relaxed
Eating and drinking Potential risk of inhaling during anaesthesia	Withhold food and drink for about six to eight hours pre-operatively, except for medications—attach 'nil by mouth' notice to the bed: ensure that the patient knows why this is necessary	Anaesthetic not complicated by inhalation of vomit
Breathing Potential risk of chest infection causing coughing and dehiscence of the incision	Practise deep breathing exercises with patient: refer to physiotherapist if necessary	Knowledgeable patient who understands why these exercises are important post-operatively

Treatment and care vary with the disorder, surgery to be performed, type of anaesthetic and the surgeon. Specific requirements are aided with discussion of the various disorders.

Table 20.3 *Specific post-operative care of patients undergoing intra-ocular surgery (continued overleaf)*

Patient's problems	Nursing intervention	Expected outcome
Potential difficulty with breathing	Maintain a clear airway and observe operations until the patient has fully recovered from the general anaesthetic	Adequate respiration with no acquired chest infection
	Encourage deep breathing exercises and sit them up in bed as soon as possible/allowed to encourage lung expansion	
	Try to avoid any situation that may cause the patient to cough; if this is not possible, teach them to cough with their mouth open	Prevention of increased intra-ocular pressure leading to the possible development of a hyphaema or prolapsed iris
Pain	Mild pain is to be expected, and relieved with suitable analgesic agents	A comfortable, pain-free patient
	Severe pain, particularly if it develops suddenly, is reported to the doctor	
Difficulty with mobilization due to: • decreased visual activity • effects of anaesthetic • being unable to bend or lift, so as not to put a strain on the incision	Rate of mobilization varies according to surgeon and progress made, but the patient should be mobilized as soon as possible, and escorted when first allowed to walk around	An increasingly mobile patient
	Encourage leg exercises and frequent changes of position	Prevention of pressure sores and deep vein thrombosis
	Keep all walking aids easily available, and ensure that the call bell is within reach—respond willingly to any request for assistance	Patient moving around confidently
	Explain the need for gentle, not jerky, sudden movements, especially of the head	No abnormal strain placed on the incision

Inability to maintain own hygiene and dress unaided	Assist with wash	Hygiene maintained
	Help in dressing; advise on suitability of clothing, avoiding clothes that have to be pulled on over the head	Dressing achieved safely
	Supply aids that allow patient to dress without bending	
Potential risk of delayed healing due to an infection	Eye dressing carried out as per procedure, and observed for any signs of infection, e.g. increased conjunctival injection, discharge or hypopyon	An uneventful recovery, without any intra-ocular complications
	Instillation of prescribed topical antibiotics	
	Ask the patient not to rub or wipe his eyes with a dirty handkerchief, or interfere with the dressing	
	Temperature to be recorded regularly, and any elevation above the norm reported	
	Eye to be protected at night by a dressing or plastic shield, to prevent inadvertent contact	
Difficulty with eating or drinking due to: • visual impairment • position in bed • effects of anaesthetic	Commence sips of water on return from theatre, then gradually build up to a light, easily digestible diet the day after, especially if the patient is being nursed flat on his back	Restoration of balanced diet to aid healing
	Encourage fluids, but decrease if the patient complains of nausea and give an anti-emetic	No rise in intra-ocular pressure due to vomiting; an intact incision
	Record fluid intake and output until the patient is capable of taking control of his own eating and drinking	Adequate fluid intake
	Assist with meals and make sure there is always a drink available in a suitable glass/feeder or with a Flexi-straw	

(cont.)

Table 20.3 (*cont.*)

Difficulty with elimination	Encourage adequate fluid intake, especially if on bed rest	Normal bowel and urinary function maintained, avoidance of constipation, a good urine output
	Advise the patient to choose a high-fibre diet; give aperients if necessary	No straining, so avoiding any rise in intra-ocular pressure
Difficulty in maintaining own safety	Re-orientate the patient to the ward on return from theatre: if he is disorientated put sides on bed and observe closely	Well-orientated patients, safe within the hospital environment
	Assess degree of orientation frequently	
	Keep call bell within easy reach, also all articles likely to be needed; always keep things in the same place	
	When mobile, keep surrounding area free of unnecessary obstruction, and all equipment/furniture should not be moved without informing the patient	
	Be aware of the importance of significant sensory input in the maintenance of orientation to time and place	
	Encourage people the patient knows well to visit	
	Try to anticipate the patient's needs	
	Inform all departments and staff, medical, nursing, paramedical and ancillary, of the patient's degree of visual handicap	
	Adjust lighting to suit the patient's requirements; once the dressing has been removed, give dark glasses	Avoidance of photophobia and the danger of consequent squeezing of the eye, raising the intra-ocular pressure
Inability to rest and sleep	Position comfortably in bed; surgery may preclude the patient's sleeping in his usual position	A relaxed, rested patient

Problem	Nursing action	Goal
	Give night sedation as required	
	Ensure that the patient does not lie on his affected side unless requested to do so	
Difficulty with communication	Communicate clearly verbally, be aware of the inadequacy of non-verbal communication for the patient with visual impairment, use tone of voice and touch rather than body movement and facial expression	Establishment of effective communication
	Approach from the better sighted side; speak before arriving at the patient's side	Make the patient aware of your presence without startling him
Boredom	Provide diversional therapy, e.g. radio or talking books	Relaxed patient for whom time passes quickly
Anxiety:		
• Outcome of surgery	Give information about outcome of surgery; ask medical staff to see the patient if necessary	Patient is confident about the result of surgery, and feels confident to return home
• Ability to cope at home	Check arrangements for convalescence; organize convalescence if necessary	
	Inform family of restrictions that still apply, e.g. no bending and no lifting	
	Demonstrate to, and observe the patient carrying out the instillation of eye medication: arrange for a district nurse to visit if there is any problem	
	Contact social worker about arranging Meals-on-Wheels and home helps if necessary/required	
	Reassure the patient as to the availability of advice; reassure him that he can phone or visit if he is worried about anything, no matter however trivial it may seem	
	Inform about length of convalescence required and reassure about the patient's ability to return to work if appropriate	Restoration of normal lifestyle

the trusting relationship that constitutes the major element of
ophthalmic nursing to both patient and nurse.

FURTHER READING

Hunt, J. & Marks-Maran, D.J. (1980) *Nursing Care Plans; The Nursing Process
at Work*. London: H.M. & M.
Kershaw, B. & Salvage, J. (1986) *Models for Nursing*. Chichester: Wiley.
McFarlane, J. & Castledine, G. (1982) *A Guide to the Practice of Nursing using
the Nursing Process*. London: C.V. Mosby.
Pearson, A. & Vaughan, B. (1986) *Nursing Models for Practice*. London: Heine-
mann.
Roper, N., Logan, W. & Tierney, A. (1985) *The Elements of Nursing*. Edinburgh:
Churchill Livingstone.

Appendix: Ophthalmic drugs

The method for administration of ophthalmic drugs in drop or ointment form is described in Chapter 2. The ophthalmic nurse must, however, acquaint herself not only with safe practice in regard to drug administration but also with the effects of the more commonly used ophthalmic medications. An understanding of the actions of the drugs which she instils will enhance her ability to prepare her patients for therapy and will ensure that any unwanted reactions are promptly noted and dealt with.

DRUGS AFFECTING THE AUTONOMIC NERVOUS SYSTEM

The intra-ocular muscles which control the pupil and accommodation are under the control of the sympathetic and parasympathetic nerves of the autonomic nervous system. Drugs can stimulate, mimic or block these systems, and cause the pupil to dilate or constrict and paralyse the muscles of accommodation.

MYDRIATICS

These drugs dilate the pupil. The plant belladonna (deadly nightshade) was used for this purpose in ancient times, as wide pupils were thought to enhance beauty.

Anticholinergic drugs

These drugs block the transmission of acetylcholine and leave the pupil under the influence only of the sympathetic nerves. This causes dilatation of the pupil and paralysis of the ciliary muscle (cycloplegia) used for accommodation. Anticholinergic mydriatics are used to aid ophthalmic examination, to rest the eye, to prevent synechiae when iritis is present and in some cases of lamellar cataract.

Atropine 1% is the most commonly used mydriatic. It is obtained from belladonna and produces mydriasis within 30 minutes. It fixes accommodation at distant focus. Its main disadvantage is that its effects persist for about 14 days and its action is not readily reversed by miotic drugs. It may cause local irritation and skin oedema.

Homatropine 1–5% is milder and less persistent. Mydriasis may persist for up to 48 hours, and it does not cause complete cycloplegia in children.

Cyclopentolate (Mydrilate) 0.5–1% has been more extensively used in recent years. Its effect lasts for only about six hours, and so repeated doses are necessary when the drug is used to rest the eye following surgery.

Tropicamide (Mydriacyl) 0.5%–1% is a rapid-acting mydriatic and cycloplegic, with a maximum effect 20 minutes after administration. The effects last for only about six hours.

Sympathomimetic drugs

These drugs stimulate the sympathetic nerve endings and produce mydriasis without cycloplegia.

Phenylephrine 2–10% is the most commonly used drug in this category. Mydriasis occurs within 20 minutes and lasts for about three hours. Phenylephrine 10% may be dangerous in eyes with shallow anterior chambers and narrow drainage angles, when it may cause acute closed angle glaucoma. The drug is commonly used with an anticholinergic agent for ophthalmoscopy, breaking down of posterior synechiae, and pre-operatively for cataract extraction.

MIOTICS

Miotics are drugs which constrict the pupil either by stimulating the parasympathetic nerve or by mimicking its action. The ciliary muscle also constricts, opening up the canal of Schlemm and allowing drainage.

Pilocarpine 0.5–4% is a moderately powerful miotic. Maximum miosis is attained in about 30 minutes and the effect persists for 10–12 hours. Intra-ocular tension is lowered for up to eight hours. Pilocarpine is used to reverse the effects of mydriatics following clinical examination and to reduce the intra-ocular pressure in glaucoma. The minimum amount of the weakest solution that will control the glaucoma is used, since side-effects (irritation on instillation, transient headache and mild spasms of accommodation) are common though rarely severe.

HYPOTENSIVE DRUGS

The drugs in this group act to reduce intra-ocular pressure by means other than miosis.

EPINEPHRYL BORATE (EPPY) 0.5% AND 1%

This drug is a sympathomimetic and acts to decrease aqueous production and increase its outflow. Miosis does not occur (this is especially desirable in patients with incipient cataract) and the effects of the drug last for 12–72 hours so it is used only once or twice daily. Side-effects are relatively common and include local allergy, headache and heart palpitations.

TIMOLOL MALEATE (TIMOPTOL) 0.25% AND 0.5%

This beta-adrenergic receptor blocking drug (beta-blocker) inhibits aqueous production without causing miosis or cycloplegia. Side-effects are rare, but the drug is powerful and should be used with caution.

CARBONIC ANHYDRASE INHIBITORS

This group of drugs acts in the ciliary body of the eye to reduce the secretion of aqueous. Acetazolamide (Diamox), methazolamide

(Neptazane) and ethoxzolamide (Cardrase) are all examples of this group of drugs, which are given in tablet form to those patients whose intra-ocular pressure cannot be controlled with drops alone. Because of the undesirable side-effects of these drugs (including potassium depletion, gastric upset, exfoliative dermatitis, renal stones, shortness of breath, tingling extremities and fatigue) these drugs are generally used only as a short-term therapy.

ANTIBIOTICS

Antibiotics are chemical substances which have the capacity, in dilute solution, to inhibit the growth of (bacteriostatic) or destroy (bactericidal) micro-organisms. In treating infections of the eye, correct diagnosis, culturing of bacteria and testing for sensitivity reactions in order to select the correct antibacterial agent are vitally important. Most of the preparations are administered topically, although systemic treatment or intra-ocular injection may be necessary for some infections. The drugs may also be used prophylactically both before and after surgery to the eye.

Chloramphenicol (Chloromycetin) is a bacteriostatic agent and is effective against a wide range of Gram positive and Gram negative organisms. It is available both in drop (0.5%) and ointment (1%) form for topical use; its systemic use is rare because of undesirable side-effects. Indications for use include conjunctivitis, blepharitis and other superficial infections. The drug is commonly used prior to and following intra-ocular surgery as a prophylactic measure.

Neomycin is a broad-spectrum bactericidal agent. It is never used systemically but may be used as eye drops or ointment (both 0.5%) and as a subconjunctival injection. It is used to treat superficial ophthalmic infections and prophylactically before and after intra-ocular surgery.

Soframycin (Framycetin) is also bactericidal against a wide range of organisms. It is available as drops (1%), ointment (0.5%) and for subconjunctival injection, and may be used to treat superficial infections or prophylactically.

Tetracyclines are a group of drugs including oxytetracycline, chlortetracycline and tetracycline itself, all of which are bacteriostatic in action. They are most commonly prescribed for topical application in ointment form, although drops are available. These drugs are also effective when taken orally. Indications for use include trachoma, conjunctivitis, blepharitis and ophthalmia neonatorum. The drugs may also be used prophylactically.

The penicillin group of drugs, polymixins and gentamicin, are also commonly used in the treatment of ophthalmic infections.

CORTICOSTEROIDS

Corticosteroids are used topically to treat inflammatory conditions of the eye, particularly uveitis, iritis, choroiditis, episcleritis, pingueculitis and chemical burns. They are also used to reduce scarring following inflammation, trauma, surgery and chemical burns, although they are used with caution in these instances since they may delay wound healing. Those most commonly used include cortisone, prednisolone, betamethasone (Betnesol), dexamethasone, hydrocortisone and methylprednisolone (Depomedrone). Topical application is effective in treating inflammation of the eyelids, conjunctiva, sclera and cornea, but subconjunctival injection may be necessary where iridocyclitis or uveitis are present. Systemic corticosteroids are indicated when the anterior segments of the eye, the orbit or the optic nerve are involved.

Corticosteroids must be used with care, and topical application may cause perforation of the cornea in the presence of infection. Secondary glaucoma is a side-effect of prolonged use of topical steroids. Systemic effects include fat redistribution, fluid retention, glycosuria and hypertension.

Glossary

Abscise To cut away, e.g. a piece of prolapsed iris.
Accommodation The ability of the lens to alter its convexity and allow near objects to be focused on the retina.
Albinism A hereditary deficiency of pigment.
Amaurosis fugax Recurrent transient loss of vision in a quiet eye.
Amblyopia Reduction of vision in an eye that appears normal.
Aniridia Congenital absence of the iris.
Anisometropia A difference in the refractive error of each eye, e.g. one eye is myopic and the other hypermetropic.
Anterior chamber This is bounded by the posterior surface of the cornea and the anterior surface of the iris. It is filled with aqueous humour.
Anterior segment of the eye This comprises the anterior and posterior chambers.
Aphakia An eye which has had its lens removed for whatever reasons.
Aqueous humour The clear fluid in the anterior chamber which is constantly secreted by the ciliary processes.
Astigmatism in the eye A refractive problem due to an irregularity of the corneal surface. The corneal meridians are unequal.

Binocular vision The ability of both eyes to focus on one object and fuse the two into one.
Blepharitis Inflammation of the eyelid margins; it may also be ulcerative.
Blepharospasm Spasm of the eyelids. There is excessive and exaggerated blinking.
Blind spot A blind area in the visual field that corresponds to the area where the nerve fibres leave the eyeball as the optic nerve.
Buphthalmos Large eyeball found in infantile glaucoma.

Canal of Schlemm A circular channel located at the limbal area of the anterior chamber. This allows for the drainage of aqueous humour.
Canaliculus Small passage from the punctum to the lacrimal sac for the drainage of tears; there is an upper and lower.
Canthus The inner and outer or medial and lateral aspect of the aperture of the eyelids.
Cartella shield A metal shield with perforations, used to protect the eye.
Caruncle The fleshy nodule at the inner canthus of the eye.
Cataract Opacity of the lens.
Chalazion Often called a meibomian cyst, it is really a granulomatous inflammation of a meibomian gland.
Chemosis Oedema of the conjunctiva.
Choroid The middle and vascular coat of the eyeball.

Cilia Eyelash.

Ciliary body The middle part of the uveal tract, comprising the ciliary muscle, which is the muscle of accommodation, and the ciliary processes which produce aqueous humour.

Coloboma A congenital defect in which there is a piece missing, e.g. a segment of the iris.

Colour blindness A decrease in the ability to see colours or, more commonly, one colour.

Commotia retinae Oedema of the retina resulting from a contusion injury to the eye.

Concave lens Known as a negative lens and indicated with a minus sign. It diverges light rays and so is used to correct myopia.

Concretions White spots caused by the gathering of degenerative or inflammatory products in the palpebral conjunctiva. May require removal if they irritate the patient's lid/eye.

Conjunctiva The mucous membrane which lines the eyelids and is then reflected onto the eyeball as far forward as the limbus.

Contact lenses Lenses that fit onto the front of the cornea.

Convergence The visual axes are directed to a near point, e.g. when reading.

Cornea The transparent window forming the anterior one-sixth of the eyeball.

Corneal graft Also known as a keratoplasty: the replacing of a piece of opaque cornea with a piece of clear cornea from a donor eye.

Cover test This test determines the presence or absence of squint.

Cycloplegic A drug that paralyses the ciliary muscle and fixes the focus of the eye for distance.

Dacryocystitis Inflammation of the lacrimal sac.

Dark adaptation The ability of the pupil and the retina to adjust to a decrease in the light.

Diopter The strength of the refractive power of lenses is measured in diopters.

Diplopia Double vision.

Discission An operation in which the anterior lens capsule is ruptured to allow soft lens matter to be absorbed or removed.

Distichiasis A double row of lashes; the abnormal row tend to turn in.

Diurnal The change in intra-ocular pressure that takes place during the night over a number of hours.

Drainage angle The area at the periphery of the anterior chamber where the drainage of aqueous humour takes place.

Ecchymosis Bruised, swollen eyelids (a 'black eye').

Ectropion A turning or rolling outwards of the eyelids.

Emmetropia Normal eyesight, where there is no refractive error.

Endogenous Coming from within.

Endophthalmitis Severe intra-ocular infection.

Entropion A turning or rolling inwards of the eyelids.

Enucleation The surgical removal of the eye, including the sclera.
Epicanthus A vertical fold of skin at the inner canthus of the eye.
Epilation The removal of eyelashes.
Epiphora The spilling over of tears.
Esophoria A tendency for the eye to turn inwards.
Esotropia An obvious or manifest turning inwards of the eye.
Evisceration Removal of the contents of the eyeball, but leaving the sclera.
Exenteration Removal of all of the contents of the orbit, including the eyeball and eyelids.
Exophoria A tendency for the eye to turn outwards.
Exophthalmos Abnormal protrusion of the eyeballs. This word is usually used when both eyes are protruding.
Exotrophia An obvious or manifest turning outwards of the eye.

Floaters Little dark portions in the vitreous: small pieces of the scaffolding of the vitreous that have broken off.
Fornix The area where the palpebral conjunctiva is reflected onto the eyeball. It forms a little pouch.
Fovea The area of acute vision, a small depression in the macula.
Fundus The posterior part of the eyeball, which can be seen with an ophthalmoscope.
Fusion The ability to coordinate the images of the two eyes into one image.

Glaucoma Abnormal rise in intra-ocular pressure.
Gonioscopy A technique to examine the drainage angle of the eye by using a contact lens with a built-in mirror and a slit lamp.
Goniotomy A surgical procedure in the treatment of buphthalmos.

Hemianopia Loss of vision in one half of the field of vision of one or both eyes.
Heterophoria A tendency of the eyes to deviate.
Heterotropia A manifest or obvious deviation of the eyes.
Hordeolum (external) Infection of the glands of Zeis (stye).
Hordeolum (internal) Infection of the meibomian gland (Chalazion).
Hypermetropia Long sight.
Hyperphoria A tendency for the eyes to deviate upwards.
Hypertropia A manifest or obvious deviation of the eye upwards.
Hyphaema Blood in the anterior chamber.
Hypopyon Pus in the anterior chamber.
Hundred Hue Test Test to elicit a colour vision defect.

Iridectomy Removal of part of the iris.
Iridocyclitis Inflammation of the iris and ciliary body, also known as anterior uveitis.
Iridodialysis Tearing of the iris from its root at the ciliary body.

Iridodonesis   A quivering of the iris, obvious in eyes that have had the lens removed.
Iris   The coloured curtain of the eye which is pierced in the centre by the pupil.
Ischaemia   Lack of blood to a part.
Ishihara Test   Test to elicit a colour vision defect.

Keratitis   Inflammation of the cornea.
Keratoconus   Abnormal cone shape of the cornea.
Keratoplasty   A corneal graft: the replacing of a piece of opaque cornea with a piece of clear cornea from a donor eye.
Keratoprosthesis   The replacing of an opaque cornea with an artificial cornea.

Lacrimal sac   The pouch at the junction of the naso-lacrimal duct and the canaliculi.
Lacrimation   Excessive production of tears.
Lamina cribrosa   Sieve-like structure and weak area of the sclera through which the optic nerve passes.
Laser   Light amplification by stimulated emission of radiation.
Lens   The focusing mechanism of the eye.
Limbus   Junction of the cornea and the sclera.

Macula lutea   The area of acute vision on the retina, surrounding the fovea centralis.
Meibomian cyst (Chalazion)   An internal hardeolum.
Meibomian glands   Little glands that are situated in the tarsal plate of the eyelids.
Microphthalmos   Abnormally small eyeballs.
Miotic   A drug that constricts the pupils.
Mydriatic   A drug that dilates the pupils.
Myopia   Short sightedness, due to a long eye.

Needling   The capsule of the lens is torn with a needle.
Nematode   A genus of worms.
Nystagmus   An involuntary rapid movement of the eyeball.

Ophthalmia neonatorum   Conjunctivitis of the newborn, and often presents with purulent discharge.
Ophthalmoscope   This instrument allows the examination of the fundus of the eye due to its special illumination system and varieties of lenses. There is a direct ophthalmoscope and an indirect ophthalmoscope. The latter allows examination of the periphery of the retina.
Optic atrophy   Degeneration of the optic nerve.
Optic cup   The central depression in the optic disc.
Optic disc   The area where the retinal fibres leave the eyeball as the optic nerve.

Optician (optometrist)   A person trained in the measurement of the refraction of the eye.

Ora serrata   The anterior boundary of the retina.

Orthoptist   A person trained in the management of extra-ocular muscle imbalance.

Oscillopsia   The sensation of objects moving, and occurs in some types of nystagmus.

Palpebral   Pertaining to the eyelid.

Palpebral fissure   The distance between the upper and lower eyelids.

Pannus   The encroachment of blood vessels onto the cornea. The term is mainly used where the corneal vessels are the result of trachoma and encroach from the superior border of the cornea.

Panophthalmitis   Generalized infection of the eye.

Paracentesis   Tapping the anterior chamber to lower the intra-ocular pressure quickly. Usually, a needle is inserted at the limbus.

Perimeter   An instrument for measuring the field of vision.

Peripheral vision   The ability to perceive an image at the side when an eye is in an undeviated straight-ahead gaze.

Photocoagulation   Through high-powered light there is a controlled burn of the choroid and retinal pigment; this in turn causes an inflammatory reaction. It is used in the treatment of retinal disorders.

Photophobia   Abnormal sensitivity to light.

Phthisis bulbi   Soft destruction of the eyeball. The eyeball shrinks.

Pinguecula   A yellow nodule that may appear on one or both sides of the cornea.

Posterior chamber   The area where the lens is suspended. It is bounded by the posterior surface of the iris and the anterior vitreous face. The ciliary processes also form a border.

Posterior segment   The vitreous cavity.

Presbyopia   Reduced power of accommodation due to advancing years.

Proptosis   Prominence of the eyeball and eyelids. This term is used mainly when one eye is prominent.

Pterygium   A triangular fold of tissue from the conjunctiva which encroaches onto the cornea.

Ptosis   A drooping of the eyelid.

Pupil   The round opening in the middle of the iris. It controls the amount of light allowed to enter the eye.

Recession   The extra-ocular muscle is cut from its insertion and re-attached posteriorly.

Refraction   The bending of light rays as they pass from one transparent medium into another of a different density.

Refractive error   Where light rays entering the eye do not focus on the retina.

Refractive media   Those transparent parts of the eye which bend light rays entering the eye.

Resection   Removal of part of a muscle.
Retina   The innermost layer of the eyeball, the light-sensitive layer.
Retinal detachment   The separation of the neural layers of the retina from the pigment epithelial layer and choroid.
Rhodopsin   Visual purple of the rod cells.
Rods and cones   The photoreceptors of the retina.

Sarcoidosis   A rare disease, in some ways similar to tuberculosis, which may affect the eye.
Sclera   The tough white outer layer of the eyeball.
Scotoma   A visual field defect.
Slit lamp   A microscope with a specialized illuminating system.
Snellen's Chart   A chart of graded sized letters for testing central visual acuity.
Stenosis   The narrowing or contracting of channels.
Strabismus (squint)   When the visual axes are no longer parallel.
Stye   External hordeolum.
Sympathetic ophthalmitis   Inflammation of an eye following traumatic inflammation of the fellow eye.
Synechia   Adhesions of the iris to the lens behind (posterior) or the cornea in front (anterior).

Tarsorrhaphy   The suturing together of the eyelids, either partly or completely.
Telangiectatic   Dilated, tortuous capillaries.
Tenon's capsule   Sheath of tissue creating a socket for the eyeball. It extends as far forward as the limbus.
Tonometer   An instrument for the measurement of intra-ocular pressure.
Trabecular meshwork   The meshwork through which the aqueous humour passes to enter the canal of Schlemm.
Trichiasis   Lashes that turn inwards against the cornea.
Trochlea   Fibrous pulley through which the superior oblique muscle passes.

Uvea (the uveal tract)   The iris, ciliary body and choroid.
Uveitis   Inflammation of part or all of the uveal tract.

Visual acuity   The faculty the eye possesses of perceiving shape or form of objects in direct vision.
Vitreous humour   The gel filling the posterior segment.

Zonule   Suspending ligament which suspends the lens.

Index